THE 4-WEEK GUT HEALTH PROTOCOL FOR BEGINNERS

A SCIENTIFIC APPROACH FOR A LEAKY GUT WITH
HOLISTIC NUTRITION TO RESTORE YOUR HEALTH
INSIDE OUT (BEST RECIPES FOR MICROBIOME
HEALTH INCLUDED)

DUNCAN PASCAL

Special Bonus

Want *Access* to the Gut Health Protocol Task Card Below?

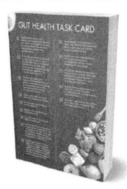

Get a *FREE*, printable version of the task list, along with early access to my new books by joining my fanbase!

Scan with your camera to join!

CONTENTS

ABOUT THE AUTHOR

In a world where seven of the leading 10 causes of death are chronic diseases, understanding the critical role of gut health has become paramount. Duncan Pascal, an author and nutrition enthusiast, has dedicated himself to educating people on the importance of maintaining a healthy gut. With a wealth of experience, he has witnessed the consequences of preventable ailments, nutrition-related health issues, and the impact of poor gut habits.

In his latest book, he unveils how we can address the root causes of these health concerns long before seeking medical intervention. Duncan advocates a holistic approach to enhancing gut health, emphasizing the significance of proper nutrition and regular exercise. He firmly believes that prioritizing gut health is the key to preventing chronic conditions such as diabetes and inflammation.

Within these pages, you will discover essential topics that include:

- Strategies encompassing diet, exercise, stress management, and integrative health practices to enhance your gut microbiome.
- Insights into digestive and gut disorders, their underlying causes, symptoms, exacerbating factors, and natural remedies for swift relief.
- Nutritional choices that promote improved gut health.
- Unveiling the truth about leaky gut syndrome and exploring natural methods to address it.
- Comprehensive information on the gut microbiota.
- A discussion on the challenges of maintaining a healthy diet.
- A collection of delightful recipes aimed at detoxification and sustaining optimal gut health.

Duncan Pascal imparts proven methods for bolstering and preserving one's health, all without the need for extravagant investments in miracle products.

INTRODUCTION

Monica's gut crisis was brutal and sudden. Six years after having her first child, she suffered joint pain, insomnia, and low libido. Like other busy moms, she thought her demanding schedule had precipitated her circumstances. Although she was mildly concerned, she believed her health would eventually improve.

Her situation showed no sign of improving, however, and Monica became worried. She was tested for Lyme infection, thyroid disorders, mononucleosis, and other potential catalysts but they all returned a negative result. Since her healthcare providers could not determine the cause of her ailment, they simply advised her to manage stress and improve her sleep.

But Monica finally found the answer she was looking for after visiting Daniella, a Colorado food expert. Daniella encouraged Monica to do a diet sensitivity blood test and create a catalog of the meals she consumed. As it turned out, Daniella was right; test outcomes showed Monica was sensitive to sugar, gluten, caffeine, dairy, and soy – everything she enjoyed eating!

If you're reading this, you probably don't understand how the gut works but are looking for a resource that offers a scientific approach to many of the theories about leaky gut and overall gut health. Maybe you've heard that an improved gut system helps prevent (or improve) immune disorders, cancer, digestive conditions, diabetes, and mental health issues, but don't know how to strengthen your beneficial stomach microbes.

Perhaps you're battling gut health issues and want to know what to do about it immediately. You've done everything to remedy nutritional deficiencies, skin irritations, headaches, widespread inflammation or chronic diarrhea, but aren't having the proper outcomes. Like Monica, the therapeutic procedures your healthcare providers have suggested have been ineffective.

Maybe you decided to follow a natural approach to improving your digestive health and sought guidance on how to do this successfully, but the natural remedies you found online were difficult to follow or never produced the results they promised. Now you feel like giving up on this journey to better gut health.

But what if someone shared with you the scientifically-based information you need to clarify your confusion about gut health and leaky gut syndrome? If someone showed you how to permanently handle your leaky gut issues once and for all, would you listen? Wouldn't you feel great if you discovered a comprehensive natural approach to gut health that merely involved a healthy diet and exercise plans?

This book will provide you with the answers to all your questions about gut health - from what foods to eat for optimal digestion, to incorporating diet and exercise into a comprehensive wellness program. Besides the tried-and-tested approaches for boosting and maintaining gut health that you will discover in this book, you will have detailed knowledge about digestive and gut disorders – their root causes, symptoms, what exacerbates them, and natural ways to relieve them within a short time.

Here's why you should read this book:

- You will discover how to pay special attention to your gut health, including the body parts that make up the gut.

- You will have a new scientific approach for fixing a leaky gut – and a better understanding of the leaky gut hypothesis and symptoms, what to believe, and root causes.

- I will show you a holistic gut health nutrition plan that incorporates practical cleansing procedures, healing and rejuvenation protocols, eating right, and exercise or movement options to strengthen gut health and general well-being.

- You will discover the best food categories for microbiome health and gut-friendly probiotics, and prebiotic recipes you can make at home.

For remedying gut-related health issues, there's no quick-fix solution for everyone because we all have different microbiome compositions. Like your fingerprints, your stomach bacteria are unique to you. So, there's no point in suggesting a diet someone else used to fix their gut issues, because it may not produce a positive outcome for you, but the detailed guide in this book will give you step-by-step instructions on how to create and maintain your own DIY gut health plan.

I have helped hundreds of people overcome issues with their gut health, particularly those with leaky gut problems. I have been studying the best methods for approaching gut health naturally for several years now. Helping you achieve freedom from complicated gut health problems is important to me because what you are about to learn helped me overcome my own struggles with these issues and become better at taking good care of myself and my digestive health.

I know how difficult it can be to absorb all the facts that pertain to gut health maintenance, but I will show you how to work things out without stress. My passion for helping people overcome their digestive problems and avoid gut-related health complications like irritable bowel syndrome, chronic inflammation, and leaky gut motivated me to write this book. I'm confident that the strategies I share with you will help you immensely, having had personal experience with these issues in the past. Understanding the gut, the microorganisms and bacteria living in our gut, and how they communicate and alter our physical and mental health is crucial to solving these lingering problems once and for all.

I wrote this book to present the information in a more comprehensible and beginner-friendly way. Often, the material available on this subject is quite academic, and therefore, may be challenging for many to grasp. I aim to offer readers an easy-to-understand resource that you can revisit time and again for guidance.

It is concerning to note the rising trend in the Western world of chronic diseases and illnesses linked to poor gut health. In the last four decades, such conditions have surged, and there is an urgent need to address this problem. We will delve into this issue further throughout this book.

Gut health is an essential aspect of overall health and well-being, so it is critical to educate ourselves and understand the crucial role it plays in our lives. With this book, I hope to empower readers with the knowledge you need to maintain a healthy gut and lead a fulfilling life.

Start your learning now, and the next time you face a gut health situation, you'll know exactly what to do. Are you ready to learn about what it'll take to get your gut health up to speed? Keep reading. Your journey to improve and restore your gut health inside-out begins *with understanding your gut*, our focus in Chapter One.

PART I

UNDERSTANDING YOUR GUT

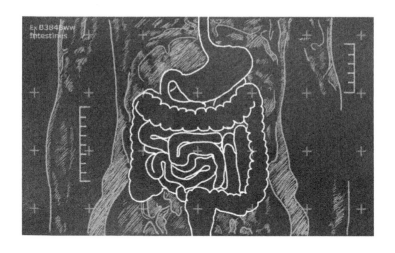

1

WHAT DOES YOUR GUT HAVE TO DO WITH ANYTHING?

Scientists researching abdomen bacteria are on the verge of making discoveries that may someday enhance the treatment of obesity, diabetes, cancer, immune syndromes, mental health ailments, and digestive disorders. The stomach bacteria in your gut are believed to be the starting point of almost all health problems, and learning how to keep it healthy could mean saying goodbye to sickness. This chapter is a comprehensive breakdown of what the gut is, its role in the human body, and why it's so important. The chapter will offer fundamental knowledge about gut health and simplify complex terminology.

What Exactly is My Gut?

Headaches. Bloating. Fatigue. Abdominal pain. Nobody wants discomforts and aches, but these are a few unpleasant consequences of gut disorder and important reasons to give your gut the attention it deserves. Your gut (also referred to as the gastrointestinal, or the GI tract – a digestive system component) is a sequence of curved organs built in an extended, twisting duct connecting the mouth to the anus (Henderson, n.d.). When we use the term microbiome or microbiota, we are referring to the community of microorganisms that live within the gut.

The gut microbiome comprises roughly 200 species of microorganisms (fungi, bacteria, and viruses) living in the digestive tract. While some microbes are toxic and lead to numerous health issues, others promote the body's metabolic activities. As we will explain throughout this book, having a diverse ecosystem of gut bacteria will help minimize psoriatic arthritis, inflammatory bowel infection, diabetes, and many other health conditions (Dix & Klein, 2022).

A person's gut health generally depends on their digestive system's bacteria varieties and levels. When there is an imbalance in the diversity or size of bacteria living within our gut, we use the term "dysbiosis" to describe this scenario. So, when you see the word "dysbiosis," just know this refers to a gut that is either a) lacking in bacterial variety or b) lacking in total number or volume of bacterial species living in the gut. Low gut bacteria diversity is considered a marker of dysbiosis.

Understanding gut health can be quite overwhelming due to the wealth of information available. Nonetheless, it is essential to grasp some fundamental concepts to make informed decisions about your gut health.

A healthy gut contains an abundance of 'good' bacteria known as gut flora. These microorganisms are present throughout our digestive system, from the mouth to the rectum. The gut flora is responsible for digesting and absorbing nutrients from our food and supporting many vital bodily functions, such as regulating our immune system. Moreover, they protect against harmful pathogens that could weaken our immune system and cause various diseases.

Conversely, an imbalance in our gut flora can result in various health conditions. Digestive issues, such as bloating, constipation, and diarrhea, are some of the most common symptoms of an unhealthy gut. Additional health problems linked to an imbalance in our gut's microbiome may include mental health conditions, obesity, and autoimmune disorders.

The science surrounding the biodiversity of the bacteria living in our gut has exploded over the last decade. Researchers can now tell if someone is overweight or fit just by looking at the diversity of the bacteria living in their gut. Understanding the science and relationship between your gut bacteria, also referred to as microbes, and your gut health is crucial to improving your overall health and preventing diseases.

The human gut is often compared to an assembly line because it is a complex system that utilizes various microorganisms to optimize the digestive process. This process is similar to a car manufacturer's assembly line, where different workers specialize in distinct tasks to improve the overall production of a product. Similarly, the gut has trillions of microorganisms, both good and bad, that have their specialized roles to perform.

Good bacteria, also referred to as probiotics, play a crucial role in the gut. They help in the breakdown of food and the absorption of vital nutrients. They also enhance the immune system and protect the gut against harmful microbes. On the other hand, harmful bacteria can be the cause of several gastrointestinal problems, such as bloating, diarrhea, and irritable bowel syndrome (IBS).

To maintain a healthy gut, a balance between good and bad bacteria is crucial. The composition of the gut's microbiome is essential to its overall health status. There are specific bacteria in the gut responsible for processing certain nutrients. For example, some bacteria break down complex carbohydrates, while others are responsible for breaking down proteins or fats. The gut also hosts bacteria responsible for producing essential vitamins like vitamin K, which aids in blood clotting, and vitamin B12, which helps maintain nerves and red blood cells' health.

The gut plays a vital role in digestion, where the nutrient extraction process takes place. The digestive system breaks down food to its molecular components to ensure that the body can absorb them and use them effectively. For instance, proteins break down into amino acids, lipids (fat and oil) break down into glycerol and fatty acids, and carbohydrates break down into sugars.

To promote a healthy microbiome, a healthy lifestyle is crucial. Consuming food that promotes healthy gut bacteria, such as fermented foods, helps support the balance of good and bad bacteria. Regular exercise programs and stress management activities also play a vital role in maintaining the stable composition of gut microbiota.

What Does My Gut Do?

The gut aids the body's optimal functioning. It facilitates the digestion process and ensures the body absorbs sufficient nutrients to thrive. From supporting skin and mental health to hormone balance, energy generation, and waste (or toxic) removal, the GI tract is crucial to the human body system (Ciccolini, 2018). Additionally, it is estimated that 70-75 percent of the immune system resides in the gut. Without a properly functioning immune system, the body is vulnerable to a wide range of infectious diseases.

Medical researchers are studying the complex significance of the gut microbiome on overall human health. Recent studies have established connections between gut health and cancer, gastrointestinal infections, autoimmune disorders, mental health, and cardiovascular ailment, but a higher gut bacteria diversity can improve our health (Dix & Klein, 2022). It appears the gut performs an incredible number of functions in our overall well-being. The gut microbiome is responsible for the following:

- **Check Bad Bacteria–** The bacteria in the GI tract multiplies rapidly, giving no room for the toxic bacteria to thrive. A healthy gut bacteria balance (technically called equilibrium) can keep you active and more vigorous. It bolsters your immune and gastrointestinal health (WebMD, 2020). Autoimmune health conditions are consequences of an imbalanced or unhealthy gut. Such situations can cause inflammation, forcing the body to attack itself.

- **Schedule Poop–** If you visit the toilet three times per day or three times a week, your poop may be normal. Each person's gut behaves differently, but a healthy GI tract follows a particular pattern. Food requires 24 and 72 hours to move through someone's digestive tract (Ciccolini, 2018). For example, it takes about eight hours for food to get to the colon, and you may feel the urge to poop afterward. Constipation can distort the poop schedule. Thyroid problems, low fiber, and dehydration are common constipation triggers, but checking your diet is an incredible way of dealing with the problem. Consuming more fruits and vegetables and drinking adequate fluids, especially water, can help.

- **Restrict Attackers–** The gut can interpret artificial sweeteners, high-fructose corn syrup, and specific processed diets as space invaders because such foods may trigger GI tract inflammation. Food absorption occurs in the GI tract, and the gut microbiome often thinks artificial ingredients are harmful. The gut activates an inflammatory response, making our body resist these foods. Consuming unprocessed meats, vegetables, fruits, and other whole foods can lessen the stress this response leaves on your body.

- **Inhibit Gluten–** Recent studies showed that gluten could accelerate intestinal permeability, commonly called the leaky gut, even when someone doesn't have a celiac disorder. A leaky gut exposes the intestine and bloodstream to pathogens and undigested food infiltration, inducing inflammation and infection (Ciccolini, 2018). Excluding gluten entirely from one's diet for four weeks (or more) and trying it again is a practical way to evaluate how their gut reacts to the ingredient. Salad dressing, chewing gum, spices, and potato chips, like many foods people consume, may contain gluten, but reading labels can help if you have a gluten-sensitive gut.

- **Improve Mental Health**– A weakened gut may increase the prevalence of depression and anxiety. Antibiotics are sometimes administered to eliminate harmful bacteria, but they often wipe out many of the gut's probiotic (helpful) bacteria as well. Some of these probiotic bacteria are instrumental in stimulating the bodies release of serotonin. Consuming prebiotics like asparagus, legumes, onions, bananas, and garlic can boost mental health.

- **Bolster Body System**– Gut probiotics keep the body active and robust. Little wonder health professionals advise people to eat kimchi, tempeh, sauerkraut, and other fermented foods that improve immune health and help the gut break down food. If you haven't been consuming fermented foods, starting with as little as 1/4 cup per serving helps prevent the digestive upset that accompanies eating more significant amounts of fermented foods.

- **Curb Sleep Disorder**– Recent studies have established a connection between a healthy gut and improved sleep, but more investigations are being conducted to verify the degree of the relationship (Ciccolini, 2018; Dix & Klein, 2022). Sufficient sleep can lessen cortisol levels and facilitate gut rehabilitation. Ensuring you sleep for seven or eight hours every night is a practical way to boost gut health and eliminate sleep disorders.

- **Hinder Stomach Upset**– Heartburn, bloating, diarrhea, and constipation are noticeable symptoms of stomach disturbances. Food processing and waste elimination difficulty often trigger these conditions. A healthy or balanced gut can eliminate stomach problems.

- **Prevent Forced Weight Modifications**– If you are accumulating or shedding weight without altering your workout habits or diet, your gut health may be compromised. An imbalanced gut can undermine nutrient absorption and disrupt fat and blood sugar regulation (Dix & Klein, 2022). Heightened inflammation and insulin resistance, and malabsorption (triggered by an imbalanced gut system) can activate weight gain and weight loss, respectively.

- **Regulate Metabolism**- Additionally, the gut can affect the production of short-chain fatty acids (SCFAs) such as butyrate, acetate, and propionate. SCFAs are produced by the fermentation of dietary fiber by gut bacteria and have been shown to play a role in regulating metabolism by promoting the release of hormones that regulate appetite, improving insulin sensitivity and reducing inflammation.

Myths and Misconceptions about Gut Health

Gut health has been extensively studied over the years. With all the misleading information online, knowing what to believe about the GI tract is fast becoming very difficult.

As researchers investigating the gut microbiome recognize the beneficial impacts of the gastrointestinal tract on the treatment of inflammatory bowel and mood disorders, gut health studies have become rampant – causing a surge in online products and blogs spreading misinformation. Let's debunk the widespread gut health myths.

- **Stress or anxiety triggers stomach ulcers**– Helicobacter pylori and other bacterial infections cause stomach ulcers, but stress and diet may aggravate the situation (Carver-Carter, n.d.).
- **Bloating is caused by what someone eats**– Many factors can trigger bloating. For example, coeliac disease (an autoimmune disorder that occurs when one's body responds to gluten), stress, and food intolerances are common bloating triggers. If you experience chronic bloating, talking to your healthcare provider may help.
- **Probiotic supplements can remedy unhealthy or leaky gut**– Consuming probiotic supplements may have health benefits, but they cannot fix leaky gut. However, since fermented foods like Miso, Kimchi, Sauerkraut, and Kombucha have high quantities of beneficial bacteria, eating them may improve gut health (Carver-Carter, n.d.). Probiotics require prebiotics to impact gut health actively, and that's why eating whole grains, fruits, and other plant-based fiber products help.
- **You must poop daily**– Nothing is wrong if you don't visit the toilet daily because normal poop is done three times daily or weekly. Factors determining how often someone uses the bathroom include stress, diet, age, and hydration levels (Carver-Carter, n.d.). Reaching out to a healthcare provider may help if there's a drastic alteration in your toilet patterns.

- **Excess fiber can unsettle the gut**– Consume about 30g of fiber daily because it can keep you active and lessen the risks of bowel cancer, heart disorder, and type 2 diabetes. Someone with a low-fiber diet should increase their intake gradually, since an abrupt rise in fiber consumption may trigger bloating (Health & Wellness, 2018).

Why Gut Health is so Important

Nausea. Abdominal pain. Constipation. Loose stools. Heartburn. Everyone suffers from these digestive disorders at some point. Persistent symptoms, however, may require medical attention. Unexpected weight loss, black stool, intense stomach aches or fever, severe throat or chest pain, jaundice, or difficulty swallowing food could be the underlying consequences of a gut disorder. If you currently experience any of these symptoms, contact your healthcare provider immediately.

The fact is, your overall health depends on your gut microbiome. There must be a balance between your digestive system's helpful and toxic bacteria before you can have a healthy gut.

The gut has a massive impact on immune function. It prevents harmful bacteria, fungi, and viruses from penetrating the bloodstream. Unfortunately, exposing the gut to threats can weaken this barrier, leading to a leaky gut and ill health. Celiac disorder, inflammatory bowel disease (IBD), and irritable bowel syndrome (IBS) are common medical conditions causing gut permeability or leaky gut (Mudge, 2022).

The gut facilitates digestion and absorbs sufficient nutrients to fuel the body. It also eliminates metabolic waste. Someone with an unhealthy gut will have trouble ridding these toxins from their body system and may experience severe fatigue, inflammation, and several chronic health complications.

To maintain a healthy gut, be prepared to deal with these factors:

- **Stress** can exacerbate intestinal permeability and trigger excess production of toxic gut bacteria.
- **Poor nutrition,** like excess consumption of sugary and processed foods, may hurt helpful gut bacteria and trigger inflammation.
- **Continual consumption of antacids and antibiotics** can eliminate the gut's beneficial bacteria. Consult your healthcare provider before using these medications (Parkview Health, 2022).

Health

Taking care of your gut health is essential for a happy and healthy life. Not only can it help you maintain a healthy weight, but there are countless other benefits as well. A healthy gut can improve digestion, regulate blood sugar levels, boost the immune system, reduce inflammation, and even improve mental clarity. All these things add up to a healthier body and mind! So don't neglect to take care of your microbiome - it's one of the most important aspects of living a balanced life.

Well-being

Furthermore, a healthy gut can be beneficial for your overall well-being. Studies show that the balance of bacteria in your gut can affect both physical and mental health. A well-balanced microbiome can help to reduce stress and anxiety, as well as improve mood and cognitive function. Not only this, but there is evidence that proper gut health may even play a role in decreasing the risk of certain diseases, such as depression, cancer and autoimmune disorders.

The latest research is beginning to acknowledge the pivotal role of gut microbiota in several physiological and pathological ways. A fascinating study published in the journal *Science Translational Medicine* in 2013 shed light on the crucial role of gut microbiota in obesity and insulin resistance. The study was centered on human twins discordant for obesity, i.e., one twin was obese while the other was lean. Transplanting the fecal microbiota from these twins into germ-free mice led to shocking findings. The mice receiving the microbiota from the obese twin displayed an abrupt increase in body fat and insulin resistance. This proves that the gut microbiota plays a vital role in regulating metabolic functions.

Furthermore, several other recent studies also suggest gut dysbiosis triggers multiple gastrointestinal disorders, such as irritable bowel syndrome (IBS). It has become apparent that maintaining a healthy gut with diverse gut microbiota composition is essential to prevent a host of health conditions. The gut microbiota significantly influences several bodily functions, such as nutrition absorption, immune system regulation, and neurotransmitter synthesis.

The importance of a healthy gut cannot be overstated, but current research findings have highlighted how little we know about our gut microbiota. By taking care of our gut, we give ourselves a better chance of preventing numerous health conditions and ensuring long-lasting health and well-being.

Is the Typical American Diet Destroying Our Gut Health?

One of the most detrimental aspects of the typical American diet is its profound impact on our microbiome. Of course, we all need food, but nowadays, it seems like the majority of us are eating processed, fatty, sugary foods that aren't doing much to nourish our bodies or support a healthy microbiome.

The convenience of processed foods has caused us to become the most obese nation in the world, and it's not just our waistlines that are suffering. Our microbiomes – which we rely on for so much – are also being negatively impacted. Five key factors show why the typical American diet is wreaking havoc on our gut health:

1. *A lack of dietary fiber* – Dietary fiber is essential for a healthy gut microbiome because it helps to promote the growth of beneficial bacteria, while also helping to regulate digestion and eliminate toxins from the body. Unfortunately, the typical American diet doesn't contain nearly enough dietary fiber, leading many people in the U.S. to suffer from digestive issues and other health problems related to their microbiome.

2. *An overabundance of simple carbohydrates and sugars* – High sugar intake has been linked with an increase in harmful bacteria in the gut, which can lead to inflammation and other negative consequences for our health. The average American consumes 22 teaspoons of added sugar each day, which is far more than the recommended daily limit of six teaspoons for women, and nine teaspoons for men.

3. *An overconsumption of processed foods* – Processed foods are notorious for their lack of fiber, vitamins, minerals and other nutrients that are essential for a healthy gut. Plus, they often contain additives such as preservatives, artificial colors and flavors that can disrupt our microbiome.

4. *A high intake of saturated fats* – This type of unhealthy fat has also been linked to obesity and other health issues, so it's important to reduce your consumption of these types of fats when possible.

5. *The effect of alcohol and caffeine* – Both alcohol and caffeine can damage the gut microbiome by increasing inflammation, negatively affecting digestion, and altering the balance of healthy bacteria. While occasional indulgences in these substances won't hugely affect our health, it's important to keep consumption within recommended limits.

The research makes it clear that the typical American diet doesn't favor our gut microbiome. One study published in the journal *Nutrients* found that diets high in processed foods, added sugars, and saturated fats were associated with decreased beneficial gut bacteria (Shi, 2019). If we want a healthy microbiome, one of the first steps is to improve our diet.

The typical American diet is unique when compared to global trends, and is causing our microbiome problems. A 2019 study looking at the diet of over 136 countries found that, on average, people in other parts of the world have a higher intake of dietary fiber and lower intake of simple carbohydrates and saturated fats than people in the U.S. (Porras & Brito, 2019).

It's no surprise, then, that gut health problems such as inflammatory bowel diseases are far more common in the U.S. than anywhere else in the world. This contrast shows how important it is for us to change our diets if we want to heal our microscopic friends and improve our gut health.

These trends correspond with the EXPLOSION of immune-mediated-based diseases over the past 50 years. This is roughly the same time period that saw the rise of industrialized food production and mass consumption of processed foods. The correlation between these two events is striking, and points to a need for us to rethink our diets if we want to take control of our health.

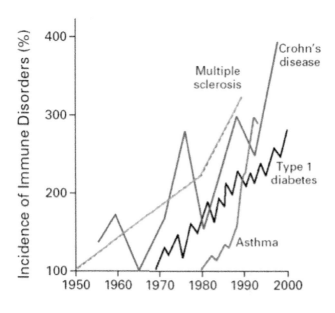

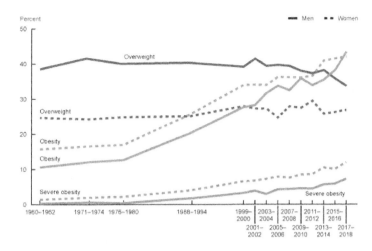

Celiac disease is up 500 percent in the past 50 years, and obesity has seen a 600 percent increase. Inflammatory bowel diseases are also on the rise, with an estimated 3 million Americans currently suffering from conditions such as ulcerative colitis and Crohn's disease. There's a relationship between gut health and many of these diseases, which points to the importance of looking after our microbiome.

Our bodies contain a complex ecosystem of microorganisms known as the human microbiome. These microorganisms are crucial for maintaining our health, helping with digestion and immune system regulation. However, the microbiome diversity of people in western countries is decreasing due to factors like antibiotic overuse, indoor lifestyles, and urbanization.

One critical factor affecting our microbiome is how we acquire it at birth. The type of delivery and feeding method at infancy can have a significant impact on the composition of our microbiome. Children born vaginally receive a richer and more diverse mix of beneficial microbes from their mother's birth canal than those delivered through a cesarean section. Additionally, breastfeeding for at least the first two years of life provides more opportunities for the transmission of healthy microorganisms from the mother. These early microorganisms can help shape a baby's developing immune system and set the stage for a healthier microbiome throughout their life.

The increasing number of cesarean deliveries in the western world is concerning, because many babies are not getting the vital early exposure to beneficial microorganisms. In the U.S., almost 33 percent of births are now by cesarean section, which suggests a worrying trend of reduced diversity in the microbiome of future generations.

Antibiotic misuse is another significant contributing factor to the decline in microbiome diversity. Particularly concerning is the overuse of antibiotics in children, which can have severe and potentially lasting effects on their gut health. Prescriptions of antibiotics for non-essential conditions or without proper follow-up measures can result in the killing of good bacteria in the gut, leading to dysbiosis - an imbalance in the microbiome - that can persist for a long time, if not addressed appropriately. Studies conducted by the Centers for Disease Control and Prevention (CDC) have revealed that at least 30 percent of antibiotic prescriptions are either not needed or are incorrect.

Exploring the Interaction Between Covid-19 and the Gut Microbiome

The COVID-19 pandemic has been a worldwide health crisis of unprecedented proportions that has had a significant impact on individuals and communities across the globe. Although the disease primarily affects the respiratory system, emerging evidence suggests that the gut microbiome may play a significant role in the progression and severity of the illness.

The gut microbiome is a complex ecosystem of trillions of microorganisms that reside within the human digestive tract. Research has shown that a diverse gut microbiome is essential for maintaining overall well being. Several studies have suggested that individuals who suffer from severe COVID-19 symptoms often have a less diverse gut microbiome than those who experience milder symptoms or remain asymptomatic.

To investigate the potential link between the gut microbiome and COVID-19 severity, a team of researchers collected blood and stool samples, as well as medical records, from 100 patients hospitalized with laboratory-confirmed COVID-19 and 78 people without the infection.

The analysis of stool samples revealed significant differences in the gut microbiome composition between infected patients and non-infected individuals, regardless of whether or not they received medication, including antibiotics. In particular, the COVID-19 patients exhibited higher levels of the species Ruminococcus gnavus, Ruminococcus torques, and Bacteroides dorei, while displaying lower levels of species that play a crucial role in influencing the immune system response, such as Bifidobacterium adolescentis, Faecalibacterium prausnitzii, and Eubacterium rectale.

Furthermore, the study found that the decreased levels of F. prausnitzii and B. bifidum were associated with an increase in disease severity, even after adjusting for age and antibiotic use. Interestingly, even after the infected patients cleared the virus from their bodies, the levels of these bacteria remained low, suggesting that COVID-19 may cause long-term alterations in the gut microbiome.

The researchers also analyzed the blood samples collected from the COVID-19 patients and found that the microbial imbalances in the gut were associated with elevated levels of inflammatory cytokines and blood markers indicative of tissue damage. This finding suggests that the gut microbiome may impact the immune system response to COVID-19 and potentially influence disease severity and outcome.

Overall, these findings strengthen the importance of maintaining a healthy and diverse gut microbiome, which may aid in the prevention and mitigation of COVID-19 and other infections.

After all, a large part of the immune system resides in the gut, so it makes sense that a healthy and diverse microbiome is essential for keeping us healthy. The good news is that there are simple steps we can all take to improve our gut health and keep our microbial friends happy.

Workbook Questions

Studying and answering these crucial questions will help you reflect on what you've learned in this chapter.

- How would you describe the gut microbiome?
- Can you specify four or five critical functions the gut performs?
- Why should someone pay attention to their gut health?
- What factors could compromise gut health well-being?

A healthy GI tract is an antidote to different medical complications, since the gut microbiome remains the starting spot for almost every health problem. The moment you begin paying attention to gut health can be the moment you bid sickness goodbye. In the next chapter, we will dig a bit deeper into the science surrounding the microbiome and its impact on our health.

2

THE AMAZING MICROBIOME

Have you ever thought of your gut as a bustling city? Just like real cities, it's home to many different citizens – but unlike human inhabitants, the citizens of your gut are microscopic. They're called the microbiome and play a critical role in our overall health and well-being.

Our microbiome consists of trillions of tiny microbes, including bacteria, viruses, fungi, and protozoa – some good, some bad. These little critters live on our surfaces, including our skin, mouth, and nose! But their biggest presence is in our digestive system; think of them as the residents in the innermost layer of this city we call "gut."

Imagine a city free of pollution and disease. That's the kind of "happy state" we strive for with our gut biome. In a healthy gut, we want to maintain a balance of good bacteria, or probiotics, which help break down food and aid in digestion, fighting off bad bacteria that can lead to diet-related illnesses, such as leaky gut syndrome.

The truth is, our guts used to be much different from what they are today. As recently as 100 years ago, humans had a very different microbiome than we have now. It has been argued that this change is due largely to industrial farming practices and over-sterilizing techniques like antibiotics, which have led to a drastic reduction in microbial diversity. In this section, we'll look at how this shift has changed how we interact with our environment and how it affects our mental and physical health.

What Exactly Is the Microbiome?

The collection of microorganisms in and on us is working to keep us healthy. It's estimated that we have trillions within our bodies and on our skin, outnumbering human cells 10 to 1!

The average size of a microbiome is about the same as two tablespoons, most of which is bacteria. The rest is made up of archaea, fungi, and viruses. Each one plays an important role in creating a healthy balance within our bodies, acting like tiny little helpers that keep us functioning optimally. The role of the microbiome is varied, but it's known to influence digestion, metabolism, immunity, and even our mood. It can also affect our skin health and the way we process vitamins and minerals.

Most of us don't realize how powerful the microbiome is for our well-being. But when it's out of balance, it can lead to various problems like digestive issues, skin conditions, and fatigue. As mentioned above, the gut microbiome is very different now from what it was even 20 years ago, and it's essential to understand this to make the right nutrition and lifestyle changes. The two main reasons for this are the modern diet, which is low in fiber and high in processed foods, and our overuse of antibiotics.

Another proposed theory for the change in the microbiome is the use of herbicides and pesticides in agriculture, which can directly impact our gut microflora. These chemicals contain some active ingredients that could be responsible for disrupting microbiome health. One ingredient that has been studied for its potential to disrupt the microbiota is glyphosate, a herbicide used in many agricultural products. Glyphosate acts by inhibiting an enzyme essential for producing certain amino acids. This can lead to inflammation, gut dysbiosis (imbalance in the composition and function of microbiota), and other health issues.

Lost microbiome species don't magically come back. Think of it as needing a certain number of Lego blocks for the roof of your house. If some are missing, the roof won't stay up. Conditions like small intestinal bacterial overgrowth (SIBO) and small intestinal fungal overgrowth (SIFO) have become more commonplace in recent decades. An estimated one in three people suffer from SIBO and SIFO (Abdulla et al., 2015).

Small intestinal bacterial overgrowth (SIBO) occurs when bacteria that should be living in the large intestine start to inhabit the small intestine, causing digestive issues such as bloating and gas. An imbalance of gut flora or an injury to the intestinal lining usually causes this. It can also be triggered by stress and poor food choices, like eating highly processed foods or a diet low in fiber. Conversely, small intestinal fungal overgrowth (SIFO) occurs when fungi that should be living in the large intestine start to inhabit the small intestine. This can also cause digestive issues and is often linked to a weakened immune system and overuse of antibiotics and other medications. It is important to understand the risks associated with SIBO and SIFO. Neglecting these conditions can result in severe health issues like malnutrition and possibly even death. It is essential to comprehend the causes and symptoms of these conditions in order to take measures to correct the imbalance in your digestive system.

The Microbiome and Your Mental Health

Many of us have already heard of the microbiome. It's been a hot topic in health and wellness circles for some time now, but most people don't know that the microbiome also plays an important role in our mental health. The mind-gut axis was first proposed by Dr. Emeran Mayer, a professor at UCLA's David Geffen School of Medicine, to explain the link between our gastrointestinal system and mental health. According to his theory, the gut-brain connection is partly mediated by the microbiome — the trillions of bacteria that live inside our gut.

The mind talks to the gut, and the gut talks to the mind. This theory has been well-researched and widely accepted, with studies showing that different mental disorders (such as depression, anxiety, and bipolar disorder) are linked to imbalances in our gut microbiome (Shoubridge et al., 2022). It's long been known that the microbiome plays a role in digestion and immunity, but its impact on mental health is only now being realized. The bacteria in your gut produce neurochemicals called neurotransmitters, which act as messengers between nerve cells. It's becoming clear that these same neurochemicals can also interact with areas of the brain involved in emotion regulation.

The link between gut bacteria and serotonin production has been studied extensively in recent years, and the findings suggest that gut health plays a crucial role in both physical and mental well-being. Serotonin, often referred to as the "feel-good" hormone, is responsible for regulating mood, appetite, and sleep, among other things. In fact, it is involved in so many bodily functions that researchers have dubbed it the "master regulator."

One of the most fascinating aspects of serotonin production is that the vast majority of it occurs in the gut rather than the brain. This means that the state of one's gut microbiome, or the collection of microorganisms that live in the digestive tract, can have a significant impact on their mood and overall health.

For example, studies have shown that people with depression and other mood disorders often have imbalances in their gut bacteria that lead to lower serotonin production. Conversely, those with a healthy and diverse gut microbiome tend to have higher levels of serotonin and are less likely to experience depression and anxiety.

Stress is a natural part of life that can arise from various situations, including work, relationships, and financial concerns. Although certain levels of stress can be motivating and helpful, prolonged exposure to stress can have adverse effects on our overall well-being. Recent research in the field of gut microbiota has unveiled a compelling connection between stress and the delicate balance of bacteria in our digestive system.

When we experience stress, the body floods the bloodstream with hormones such as cortisol and adrenaline to prime for a "fight or flight" response. These hormones have a direct impact on the balance of bacteria in our gut microflora. Studies have found that an imbalance in gut microbiota can result in inflammation, which can open the doors to an array of negative health consequences.

Additionally, the microbial strains in our gut can affect the production of neurotransmitters that regulate mood and stress levels. For instance, an increase in Bacteroidetes and a decrease in Firmicutes, two bacterial phyla, have been linked to depression and anxiety. Moreover, the amount of lactobacilli in our gut has been correlated with lower cortisol levels and reduced sensitivity to stressful stimuli. In other words, a diverse and balanced microbiome can help mitigate the impacts of stress on our mental and physical health.

When we experience prolonged periods of stress, cortisol levels can remain elevated, which disturbs the microbial balance in our gut. This imbalance, in turn, exacerbates the production of cortisol and creates a vicious cycle of psychological distress and physical discomfort.

Another convincing theory on the mind-gut connection is that the microbiome affects our mental health through its effect on inflammation. Our microbiota constantly interacts with the immune system, and it's thought that an imbalance of bacteria can trigger chronic inflammation in the body. Chronic inflammation has been linked to depression and other mental illnesses.

The incidence of common mental health disorders is increasing at an alarming rate, and it's becoming more apparent that the microbiome plays a role in this increased prevalence. Our cravings, emotional state, and even some decision-making can be traced back to our gut biology. It's clear that the microbiome is essential not only for our physical health but also for our mental well-being. If the quality of our microbiome goes awry, so will our health and happiness.

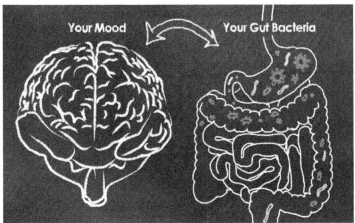

The Microbiome and Your Physical Health

Not just the mental health, but the physical health too!

The microbiome does much more than regulate our mental states - it also affects how healthy and fit we are. Our gut bacteria can affect digestion, metabolism, hormones, and even immunity. The healthier our gut microbiome is in our body, the better our overall physical health. Recent studies have shed light on how the composition of our microbiome can significantly influence our daily habits in terms of sleep, exercise, and eating patterns.

In terms of sleep, researchers have found that our gut microbiome may be able to regulate the production of sleep-related hormones like melatonin. They have discovered that certain types of bacteria can promote the production of these hormones, leading to improved sleep quality and duration. In contrast, an imbalance of gut bacteria can disrupt our circadian rhythm, resulting in sleep disturbances and insomnia.

The impact of the gut microbiome on human health is a topic of growing interest in scientific research, with numerous studies highlighting its critical role in regulating energy homeostasis and overall physiological functioning.

One area that has received particular attention is exercise.

Recent research suggests that low-intensity exercise can have a beneficial impact on gut physiology, reducing the amount of time that pathogens spend in contact with the gastrointestinal mucus layer and thereby reducing the risk of conditions such as colon cancer, diverticulosis, and inflammatory bowel disease. In addition, even in the presence of a high-fat diet, exercise has been found to reduce inflammatory infiltrate and protect intestinal morphology and integrity. Moreover, research has shown that exercising can boost the quantity of beneficial microorganisms, promote diversity among the microorganisms residing in our bodies, and improve the growth of good bacteria.

However, it is important to note that the type and intensity of exercise can also have negative effects on the gut. Endurance exercise, for example, has been found to reduce splenic blood flow by up to 80 percent, potentially leading to toxicity effects. This reduction in blood flow is due to an increase in arterial resistance in the splanchnic vascular bed, which is caused by an augmentation of sympathetic nervous system input. Additionally, prolonged exercise has been associated with increased intestinal permeability, which can compromise gut barrier function and lead to bacterial translocation from the colon.

We all know that what we eat affects us physically - if you eat unhealthy food, you're likely to gain weight, feel sluggish, and develop other ailments, such as diabetes and heart disease. But did you know that your microbiome also has something to do with this? Evidence suggests that having an entire ecosystem of healthy bacteria helps ensure better digestion of nutrients from your food, and thus, better overall physical health.

Moreover, our gut microbiome also influences our appetite and food cravings. A healthy microbial community in our gut can produce short-chain fatty acids (SCFAs) that signal to our brain that we are full and satiated. In contrast, an imbalance of gut bacteria may lead to increased hunger and cravings for unhealthy foods, contributing to weight gain and poor dietary choices.

Studies have also shown that an unhealthy microbiome is linked to obesity and other metabolic disorders, such as diabetes. An unhealthy gut flora can lead to inflammation in the body, which can cause many diseases we associate with a poor diet. The healthier the bacteria in your gut, the better chance you have of avoiding these chronic conditions.

The same goes for our immunity - having a healthy microbiome helps us fight off infection and disease more effectively than if it was unhealthy or unbalanced. Research suggests that probiotics (live bacteria found in some foods) can help strengthen immunity by boosting levels of beneficial bacteria in our bodies, thus helping us stay healthy for longer periods (Ashraf & Shah, 2014).

The impact on our hormones and why it's so crucial to have a healthy gut is a subject not discussed often enough. The microbiome plays a role in the production of hormones that are essential to our overall health, including those related to appetite, sugar metabolism, and mood. The main hormones identified with direct links to hormonal changes are:

- *Thyroid* - The microbiome can influence the production of T3 and T4 hormones, which are essential in regulating metabolism. The role is identified as participatory in the production of thyroid hormones. Disruption of the microbiome's balance can lead to a decrease of thyroid hormones and metabolic dysfunction.

- *Cortisol* - Studies have shown that the composition of our microbial population is related to how our bodies respond to stress-related hormones like cortisol (Foster et al., 2017). It appears that having a healthy gut microbiota helps reduce the secretion of cortisol and thus improves our overall mental health and physiological responses to stressful situations.

- *Estrogen* - Estrogen is a hormone important for women's health and reproduction. Studies have shown that the microbiota in our gut can influence the production of estrogen, which can affect fertility, metabolism and overall health (Lephart & Naftolin, 2022). The direct impact of the microbiome on estrogen production is still being studied, but having a healthy gut flora can help maintain balanced hormone levels.

- *Melatonin* - The microbiome also regulates the sleep-regulating hormone melatonin. Studies have demonstrated that beneficial bacteria can help regulate the production of melatonin, which helps us stay asleep and leads to better quality sleep (Zhang et al., 2022). Insomnia, which is more prevalent today than in the past, can partly be attributed to an unhealthy gut microbiome.

- *Oxytocin* - Rightly called the "love hormone," oxytocin is an important neurotransmitter that contributes to social bonding. The link between the microbiome and oxytocin production has long been established, with studies showing a direct correlation between gut health and mood-related hormones like oxytocin (Erdman, 2021). A decrease in oxytocin is linked to social isolation, anxiety, and depression.

While the derangement (disruption) of the microbiome can be linked to many health issues, restoration yields benefits far beyond gut health and bodily functions. "L. Reuteri," a bacteria considered nearly extinct today, has been shown to have astounding restorative effects in terms of both physical and mental health. From our hormones to our immunity, the impact of the microbiome on our bodies is immense and should not be underestimated.

The Microbiome and Your Immune System

The intricate connection between our gut microbiome and the strength of our immune system cannot be overstated. Research has established that these two systems work in tandem, with the gut microbiome acting as a critical regulator of the immune system's response to bacterial and viral infections.

The gut immune system is particularly active in the small intestine, where it plays an important role in preventing harmful microbes and pathogens from entering our bloodstream and vital organs. This is achieved through a complex response mechanism that involves the release of antibodies and the activation of immune cells that work together to combat any foreign invaders.

The gut microbiome's role in influencing the immune system's response cannot be overstated. Scientific evidence suggests that gut bacteria can communicate with the immune system, helping to regulate its response to infections and other health conditions. A healthy microbiome can strengthen the immune system, while a poorly maintained one can weaken it, making us more susceptible to infections and diseases.

Furthermore, metabolic and inflammatory diseases, which are prevalent in our modern age, have also been linked to the gut microbiome. Studies have shown that altering the microbiome can fundamentally change how the immune system operates, reducing the risk of chronic health conditions.

Maintaining a diverse and balanced gut microbiome that supports our immune system's strength can be achieved by consuming a healthy diet that is rich in fiber, fermented foods, and beneficial bacteria. Avoiding certain types of food, such as processed foods, can also help maintain a healthy microbiome, leading to a robust immune system that is fortified against diseases and infections.

To sum up, the connection between the strength of our immune system and our gut microbiome is intricate and interrelated. By prioritizing gut health and maintaining a healthy microbiome, we can support our immune system's strength, leading to better overall health and reduced risk of chronic health conditions.

The Microbiome and Metabolism

Our microbiome plays an important role in our metabolic health, as well. The microbiome-particular gut bacteria have a dominant role in influencing how our bodies absorb and use nutrients as well as how we store fats. Each of us has a unique microbiome, and it is now understood that the composition of our gut microflora is influenced by our genetics, diet, stress, antibiotic use, and other environmental factors.

Numerous studies have shown that a healthy microbiome can have a significant impact on metabolic health. Dr. Rob Knight, professor at the University of California, San Diego and co-founder of the Earth Microbiome Project, performed a study on triplets who developed different microbial compositions as a result of their mother's diet; their composition was primarily determined by transference of the mother's microbes during childbirth. Further studies confirmed that an individual's microbiome is specific to their lifestyle, including diet, exercise routine, and sleep patterns.

As for antibiotics, Dr. Patrice Cani's research on the effects of antibiotics on the metabolic health of humans and animals has revealed how the eradication of gut bacteria can significantly worsen metabolic health. After completing a course of antibiotics, participants showed significant alterations associated with insulin resistance and type-2 diabetes in their gut microbial composition. Additionally, testing on mice that received antibiotics revealed higher levels of glucose in their bloodstream, and this remained evident even a year after the antibiotic intervention.

Consistently incorporating healthy food choices and prebiotics, such as fiber, has been seen to promote the growth and nourishment of microorganisms for a healthier, more robust microbiome. Such practices will guarantee a healthy biome and, in turn, enhance optimal metabolic health.

The Good, Bad & Ugly Microorganisms Living in Our Gut

There are both good and bad guys among the billions of organisms in our gut. The "good" ones are beneficial probiotics linked to helping with digestion, absorbing nutrients, boosting immunity and even mood regulation. On the flip side, there are also "bad" bacteria like Candida which can wreak havoc on your digestive system if it grows out of control.

Candida is a type of yeast that resides naturally in our body, mainly in the mouth and intestines. It's normally kept under control by healthy bacteria in our body. However, when the balance is disrupted and the fungus starts to grow unchecked, it can lead to a wide range of health issues.

Let's go over some of these microorganisms and see how they affect us. We'll start with the good guys, as these are arguably the most important to our gut health and overall well-being.

The Good Guys: Probiotics

Probiotics are a type of beneficial bacteria found in fermented foods like yogurt, kimchi and sauerkraut. These helpful organisms help break down food so you can extract nutrients from it more easily and populate your intestines so bad bacteria don't get a foothold. Probiotics also play an important role in producing vitamins and enzymes essential for proper digestion.

- *L. Reuteri and L. Casei* - popular for stress, sleep management, and digestion

- *Bifidobacteria* - essential for digesting dairy and helping us absorb vitamins like B12

- *Saccharomyces boulardii* - helps reduce the risk of diarrhea and other digestive issues caused by antibiotics

The Bad Guy: Candida

Candida is a type of yeast that can cause various health problems if it gets out of balance in your gut. Beneficial bacteria usually control it, but antibiotics or dietary changes can sometimes throw off its delicate balance. Symptoms include bloating, constipation or diarrhea, fatigue, sugar cravings and more. Keeping your probiotics levels high will help keep Candida at bay!

Some bacteria don't fall into either category.

The Ugly: H. Pylori

H. pylori is a type of bacteria found in your stomach that can cause gastritis and ulcers. It's not always bad, and in some cases it may actually be beneficial - but if it becomes too plentiful, it can lead to digestive issues like gas, bloating and abdominal pain. There are treatments available for H. pylori because if left unchecked it can become dangerous.

Hopefully this has given you a better understanding of the microorganisms that live in our gut, since knowing which bacteria live there and how they interact with each other is key to maintaining optimal gut health.

The Hygiene Hypothesis

The hygiene hypothesis is a fascinating theory that has gained traction in recent years. It suggests that our immune system requires exposure to bacteria and other microorganisms early in life, and that without this exposure, the immune system may become confused and overreact to harmless substances, leading to chronic inflammation, allergies, and autoimmune disorders.

Several studies have linked the rise of allergies and autoimmune diseases to our increasingly clean and sanitized living environment. For instance, research conducted in Germany revealed that children raised on farms had lower allergy and asthma rates than those living in urban areas. The reason behind this disparity can be attributed to farm children's exposure to a more extensive range of microorganisms—especially bacteria and viruses from animals, soil, and other environmental sources—that help to train their immune systems.

Similarly, other studies have demonstrated that exposure to pets, daycare, and playing in the dirt can help reduce the likelihood of allergies and autoimmune disorders in children. These activities provide opportunities for exposure to different microbes and the development of a more robust immune system that can distinguish between friend and foe.

The balance between hygiene and exposure to bacteria and other microorganisms is key. While proper hygiene practices are essential for disease prevention, excessive use of hand sanitizers and antibiotics can have unintended consequences. Such practices can deplete the natural microbiome that resides in and on our bodies, leading to many health problems.

Workbook Questions

The following questions will help you determine if you fully understand the amazing microbiome:

- What is the relationship between the microbiome and gut health?
- What benefits do you get from having a healthy microbiome?
- How does diet influence the composition of our microbiome?
- Name two ways to support your microbiome for optimal gut health.
- Why is it important to understand how our environment affects our microbes?

- What can people do to maintain a strong and diverse microbial community in their bodies?

Now that you have a better understanding of the amazing microbiome, let's move on to methods to check the condition of your gut health. We'll be discussing how to assess your current gut health and make meaningful changes that will help you optimize it.

3

CHECKING YOUR GUT HEALTH

A re you curious about your gut health? If so, this chapter will provide you with the tools and knowledge to ensure your gut health is at its best.

While GI disorders can cause discomfort, the good news is that there are steps you can take to maintain a healthy gut. Eating a balanced diet rich in fiber and probiotics can help promote a healthy digestive system, while regular exercise can aid in the regulation of bowel movements.

It's also important to pay attention to any symptoms you may be experiencing. While nausea, bloating, and bowel movement difficulty may be signs of a GI disorder, they can also be caused by other factors. By seeking an accurate diagnosis and proper treatment, you can easily manage any issues and feel your best.

This chapter provides you with information and strategies to take control of your gut health and improve your overall quality of life. Get ready to dive in and learn how to maintain a happy and healthy digestive system!

Functional Versus Structural Gastrointestinal Diseases

GI syndromes have two forms – functional and structural. When your GI tract malfunctions with no structural abnormalities, you have FGIDs (functional gastrointestinal disorders). Infant colic, chest pain, diarrhea, and dyspepsia are all instances of active GI diseases. Structural GI disorders emanate from GI tract anomalies and may include medical conditions like colon cancer, diverticulitis, anal fistulas, ulcerative colitis, Crohn's disease, and hemorrhoids (Ambarasu, 2020).

About 40 percent of the global population has FGIDs, although the GI disorder is more widespread in women, a 2021 study confirmed. It can impact the intestines, abdomen, esophagus, or other GI tract organs (Silver, 2022). Children, adolescents, and adults can experience FGIDs, also called gut-brain interaction syndromes. A certified healthcare provider can diagnose FGID and recommend the appropriate treatment or management plan. Common conditions healthcare providers interpret as FGIDs include fecal incontinence, irritable bowel disorder, diarrhea, gastroesophageal reflux infection, constipation, indigestion (functional dyspepsia), abdominal irritation, and nausea.

Stress, smoking, and lifestyle modifications are common triggers of FGIDs, but other catalysts, such as gut sensitivity, depression or anxiety, immune system functioning, rapid or sluggish GI movements, and family history are often beyond control.

Physical symptoms of FGIDs, according to a 2017 study, include swallowing problems, abdominal discomfort, nausea, burping, flatulence, bloating, diarrhea, and indigestion, but what someone experiences depends on their condition. One 2020 FGIDs and mental health study found that depression, anxiety, and stress could exacerbate FGID symptoms (Silver, 2022).

Unlike structural GI disorders that require surgery, lifestyle changes can remedy functional GI problems. For example, healthcare providers may recommend a fiber-rich diet or workout program for FGID Patients (Clark, n.d.). Learning there's a physical defect in your digestive system could be terrifying, but a qualified GI surgeon can diagnose, discover, and fix the problem.

Without treatment, however, gastrointestinal disorders can force you to skip school, work, or any number of other important appointments. Treatment may include psychologists, therapists, counselors, dietitians, nurses, or even doctors. Of course, healthcare providers make diagnoses based on symptoms before determining the treatment. Consultation with a doctor may include these processes:

- **Interview**: Your doctor may ask about your family health record, health history, and symptoms. Answers to the questions will factor in to the treatments recommended.
- **Physical Examination**: The doctor may recommend blood, urine, and stool laboratory tests. They may also suggest you undergo a CT scan or X-ray.

Questions to expect when consulting your healthcare provider may include:

- When did you start experiencing the symptoms?
- Do these symptoms hinder you from performing any tasks?
- What foods do you eat regularly?
- Are you worried about what this ailment could be?
- What method of treatment would you prefer (oral or injection)?

Gastroesophageal Reflux Disorder

You may live with GERD (gastroesophageal reflux disease) if stomach acid often flows into your esophagus. GERD acid reflux reactions can be mild, moderate, or severe, although many people experience the problem once or twice weekly. Treatment depends on complications, but healthcare providers recommend lifestyle revisions and over-the-counter drugs for mild and moderate GERD patients. Severe conditions may require surgery or particular therapy (Mayo Clinic, 2020).

Prominent GERD symptoms include swallowing difficulty, food (or liquid) regulation, heartburn, and chest pain. People with nighttime acid reflux may suffer disrupted sleep, laryngitis, chronic cough, and asthma.

GERD occurs when belly acid streams into a person's esophagus. When you eat or drink, for example, your esophagus muscle relaxes so that the swallowed substance can move into your stomach, and the sphincter shuts. If someone's sphincter opens or is weakened, they will experience GERD. Smoking, alcohol, coffee, and late-night eating are a few factors that could exacerbate acid reflux.

Consuming a large meal may speed up acid reflux. Certain foods or sleeping after eating may also cause GERD. Common factors prompting the medical condition, according to MacGill (2022), include:

- **Obesity**: Overweight individuals experience heightened abdomen pressure. The tension forces stomach acid into the esophagus.

- **Pregnancy**: Roughly 50 percent of pregnant women suffer GERD during pregnancy.

- **Pills**: Asthma drugs, antidepressants, sedatives, and antihistamines, like many other medications, are GERD catalysts.

- **Cigarettes**: If you smoke (or regularly inhale secondhand smoke), you may experience a health condition.

GERD can trigger chronic inflammation in the esophagus, causing the following health issues:

- **Esophageal Stricture–** A point is reached in which the stomach acid harms the lower esophagus, making scar tissue grow in the food pathway. Swallowing problems become inevitable.

- **Esophageal Ulcer–** As the stomach acid weakens the esophagus tissue, an open sore develops. If you have an esophageal ulcer, you may experience bleeding, discomfort, and swallowing complications.

- **Barrett's Esophagus–** Stomach acid can damage your lower esophagus tissue lining. The stomach acid's effects on the esophagus could even heighten the risk of esophageal cancer (Mayo Clinic, 2020).

- **Respiratory Issues–** If someone inhales stomach acid into their lungs, they may experience respiratory problems like pneumonia, chest congestion, laryngitis, or asthma. For example, the findings of a 2021 study showed that GERD could facilitate the growth of idiopathic pulmonary fibrosis (MacGill, 2022). Consult your doctor for a proper diagnosis if you experience GERD symptoms.

Diagnosis may necessitate any of these tests:

- **Esophageal pH** monitors esophageal impedance and measures acid in someone's esophagus.

- **Upper GI Endoscope** is a camera tube that inspects the esophagus to determine if there is any tissue blocking the food path.

- **Upper GI Series** is an X-ray that reveals esophageal abnormalities that could cause GERD.

- **Esophageal Manometry** measures esophagus muscle construction during swallowing, including the sphincter vitality.

Since GERD is a chronic ailment, it often requires long-term supervision. Some healthcare providers suggest lifestyle changes (like avoiding food triggers, modifying diet, shedding weight, and abstaining from late-night meals), while others use medications to treat the disease (MacGill, 2022). If treatment doesn't produce a meaningful outcome, the provider may recommend surgery.

Should you experience shortness of breath, chest discomfort, or arm (or jaw) pain, seek immediate medical attention because these symptoms could be heart attack triggers (Mayo Clinic, 2020).

Lactose Intolerance

If consuming sugary foods or dairy products causes you to develop diarrhea or bloating because your body system cannot fully digest lactose, you may be living with lactose intolerance, also known as lactose malabsorption. The small intestine produces lactase, the enzyme that stimulates lactose absorption. Lactase ensures that lactose (milk sugar) turns into glucose and galactose before the intestine lining absorbs them into the bloodstream. Inadequate production of this enzyme causes lactose intolerance (Mayo Clinic, 2022).

When a lactase-deficient person consumes milk sugar, lactose penetrates their colon and reacts with the colon's bacteria to provoke lactose intolerance symptoms. Lactose intolerance has two major forms – primary and secondary.

- **Primary Lactose Intolerance**: Infants who derive their entire nutrition from breast milk produce enough lactase. But as children grow and their demand for breast milk decreases because they are consuming other foods, their lactase production also decreases. As we reach adulthood, there is a drastic decrease in lactase production.

- **Secondary Lactose Intolerance**: If someone is sick or injured, their small intestine may produce insufficient lactase. If they undergo surgery, lactase production may drop. Crohn's disorder, celiac disease, and intestinal infection are common secondary lactose intolerance health complications.

Common symptoms of lactose intolerance include nausea, diarrhea, gas, bloating, and stomach cramps. A lactose intolerant person may experience these signs 30 minutes after consuming lactose foods or beverages. For some individuals, it takes two hours for symptoms to manifest.

Lactase deficiency can cause lactose intolerance. Digestive disorders like celiac disease and ulcerative colitis can trigger the condition. Stomach infections and small intestine pains (maybe because of chemotherapy or surgery) are also common catalysts (Cleveland Clinic, 2019). Lactose intolerance risk factors include:

- **Age**: Children rarely experience lactose intolerance. The condition primarily affects adults.
- **Ethnicity**: The condition is quite common among Asian, American-Indian, African, and Hispanic people.
- **Premature Birth**: Lactase-producing cells in the small intestine develop late in the third trimester, so premature infants may develop

lactose intolerance.

- **Disease**: Crohn's disease, celiac disorder, and bacteria overgrowth, like many small intestine diseases, can hinder lactase production.

When diagnosing lactose intolerance, your healthcare provider will likely ask about your family health history. They may also conduct a physical examination. You may be told to avoid milk products for a particular period to see if that improves your symptoms (Johns Hopkins, n.d.). Lactose intolerance tests you may need to take include:

- **The stool acidity test** checks the quantity of acid in the stool. If one's stool has glucose, lactic acid, or other fatty acids, they aren't digesting lactose. A stool acidity test is carried out on babies and young children.
- **The hydrogen breath test** evaluates a person's breath after they've consumed lactose-rich liquid. If their breath contains high hydrogen levels, they are lactose intolerant.
- **The lactose tolerance test** examines how someone's digestive system digests lactose. If the test is recommended, your healthcare provider will instruct you to avoid food or drink for eight hours beforehand.

After drinking lactose-rich liquid and waiting for two hours (for digestion to occur), your healthcare provider will collect your blood sample to evaluate your blood sugar level. A rising sugar level suggests you are not lactose intolerant (Johns Hopkins, n.d.).

Diarrhea

While worldwide diarrhea cases hit two billion yearly, the medical condition annually kills roughly 1.9 million children under the age of five in developing countries. Diarrhea can be life-threatening if it is not correctly diagnosed and treated (MacGill, 2020). Watery stools may characterize diarrhea resulting from bacteria or virus infections. Digestive system syndromes may precipitate chronic diarrhea.

Diarrhea symptoms include stomach discomfort, chills, fever, and abdominal cramps. Others are body aches, weight loss, and bloating.

Common diarrhea-causing bacteria in the U.S. include Shigella, Campylobacter, Salmonella, and Escherichia coli. Technically, diarrhea comes in two forms – functional and chronic. If you display diarrhea symptoms with no digestive organ abnormalities, you have functional diarrhea. While IBS (irritable bowel syndrome) is a common active diarrhea trigger, chronic diarrhea may stem from IBD (inflammatory bowel disease). Other chronic diarrhea catalysts include:

- **Microscopic colitis,** a lasting diarrhea category in older adults, often causes inflammation.
- **Maldigestive diarrhea,** like celiac disorder, is caused by impaired digestive functioning or nutrient absorption.
- **Drug-induced diarrhea,** drugs, and laxatives side effects may occur after someone ingests antibiotics.
- **Endocrine-related diarrhea** may be caused by hormonal changes, carcinoids, and Addison's disease.
- **Neoplastic diarrhea** is a common problem in individuals with gut cancers.

Alcohol misuse, food allergies, and diabetes may also cause diarrhea (Shroff, 2021).

Proper diagnosis and treatment can help prevent the underlying conditions that diarrhea may trigger. Your healthcare provider will ask a few questions before recommending appropriate medication. Questions will focus on your current medications, medical record, family, and travel history. They may also want to know whether your stool contains blood, pus, or mucus. They may also suggest you undergo one or more of these tests:

- **Blood count** ascertains whether someone has bleeding ulcerations or malnutrition issues.
- **Malabsorption tests** screen folate, vitamin B-12, and calcium absorption and evaluate thyroid function and iron status.
- **Antibody tests** detect celiac disorder.
- **Stool tests** check parasites, viruses, or bacteria in the stool.

Mild diarrhea may not require a procedure. If an individual reports chronic diarrhea, a healthcare provider will analyze underlying causes and symptoms before suggesting medication. Treatment options include:

- **Rehydration:** Children and seniors often experience dehydration. Rehydration is usually recommended for all diarrhea cases. Drinking more fluids replenishes the body and replaces the electrolytes and water lost in watery stools. An individual with a persistent condition may require intravenous fluids.
- **Antidiarrheal Medication:** Imodium and Pepto-Bismol are common diarrhea over-the-counter drugs. Both drugs lessen watery stool

passage.

- **Antibiotics:** Bacteria-related diarrhea can be treated with antibiotics but consult your healthcare professional before taking any medications.

Food Poisoning

Anyone who consumes spoiled or contaminated food may contract a food-borne disease, typically known as food poisoning. Forty-eight million Americans experience food poisoning annually, and 128,000 are hospitalized, according to the CDC (Centers for Disease Control and Prevention) (Selner, 2021).

An individual may contract food poisoning without knowing it, but common food-borne disease symptoms include headache, fatigue, abdominal cramps, mild fever, nausea, appetite loss, vomiting, and diarrhea. Symptoms often show up 30 minutes after eating contaminated foods.

Significant causes of food poisoning are parasites, viruses, and bacteria. Although our food contains these pathogens, heat from cooking ensures they are eliminated before we serve or consume our meals. Foods that do not undergo the cooking phase often expose people to food-borne ailments. Disease-causing organisms can contaminate eggs, meat, dairy products, and even water (Selner, 2021).

Doctors consider symptoms when diagnosing food poisoning type. Your healthcare provider may ask you to provide information about how and when the ailment started. These tests can aid their diagnosis:

- **Physical examinations** like temperature, pulse rate, and blood pressure may be conducted to understand the patient's symptoms. For example, dry mouth and sunken eyes are clinical signs of dehydration (Wedro, 2022).
- **Blood tests** may be conducted when a patient suffers chronic diarrhea and vomiting. A healthcare provider may check kidney function and electrolyte levels via a blood test.
- **Stool samples** can show Salmonella, Campylobacter, and Shigella infections in patients with bloodstained stools.

Common food poisoning treatments include:

- **Proper Hydration**– Drinking sports drinks can help when someone suffers from food poisoning. If you feel weak or tired, drinking coconut water or fruit juice can help. Drinking dandelion, peppermint, chamomile, or any decaffeinated teas may soothe stomach upset.

- **OTC (over-the-counter) Drugs**– Pepto-Bismol or loperamide can calm nausea and diarrhea. It's often best to seek medical advice before taking OTC drugs.
- **Rest**– If you suffer from mild food poisoning, take a nap.

Nobody is immune from food-borne diseases, but some people (like those below) have a higher risk.

- **Immunocompromised People**: If you have an autoimmune disorder, your food poisoning infection and complication risks are high.
- **Older Adults**: If you are 65 or older, you may contract food-borne disease since your immune system may not quickly combat infectious organisms.
- **Children**: The immune system of a five-year-old is not yet fully developed. Children under five often suffer diarrhea and dehydration (Selner, 2021).

Colorectal Cancer

Cells form lines around the colon and rectum, but these cells may experience abnormal growth. When this happens, colorectal cancer develops. Undergoing regular cancer checks can help prevent such cancers, since symptoms may not show until the cancer has become advanced. Colorectal cancer risk factors include smoking, inflammatory bowel disorder, alcohol misuse, and diet (Cleveland, 2020).

Detecting colorectal cancer is complicated, since it doesn't show early-stage symptoms. However, these signs may suggest colorectal cancer:

- **Bowel Habit Changes**– If you experience bowel incontinence, diarrhea, stool narrowing, or constipation, consulting a healthcare provider may help, because these are common colorectal cancer symptoms.
- **Bloodstained Stool**– Crohn's disease, ulcerative colitis, and hemorrhoids, like many related health conditions, may trigger bleeding in the GI tract or cause bloodstained stool. Reaching out for medical help is crucial because this could also mean you're developing colorectal cancer (Cleveland, 2020).
- **Sudden Anemia**– The red blood cells ensure that your body gets adequate oxygen. Anemia occurs when there's a depletion of red

blood cells. Shortness of breath, unexplained weight loss, pelvic pain, and severe fatigue are common signs of anemia.

Healthcare providers may diagnose colorectal cancer via symptoms or examinations. Your doctor may recommend these tests during the diagnosis phase:

- Blood tests, especially tumor markers, blood count, or liver enzymes
- Angiography, ultrasound, X-rays, PET scan, CT scan, or other imaging tests
- Regular screening assessment before or after symptoms appear

Colorectal cancer treatment options include radiation, chemotherapy, and surgery. The procedure depends on the severity of the condition. Anyone may develop colorectal cancer, but these factors may put one at risk of developing the medical condition:

- **Age**: People over 50 have a higher risk of contracting colorectal cancer than younger people (Cleveland Clinic, 2020).
- **Medical Conditions**: Type 2 diabetic patients may develop colorectal cancer. People with primary cancer or inflammatory bowel disorder history also have higher risks of contracting this cancer.
- **Lifestyle**: Abuse of tobacco or alcohol can lead to the development of colorectal cancer. Fat and calorie-rich diets devoid of (or low in) fruits, fiber, and vegetables can also put one at higher risks.

Strictures

The urethra plays an extraordinary role in our overall well-being. Through this tube, both urine and semen are conveyed out of the body. Urethra strictures occur when this tube suffers an injury, infection, or swelling (Urology Care, n.d.).

Since men have a longer urethra, they have a higher risk than women of experiencing urethra strictures or infection. Common causes of strictures include urethra infection, injury, surgical damage, and swelling. Others are perineum pain, urinary catheterization, and prostate surgery.

Individuals with urethra strictures experience symptoms like abdominal discomfort, sluggish urine stream, urethra leaking, and bloody urine. Chronic urethra blockage may cause kidney trauma.

If you experience any of these symptoms or think you have urethra problems, call your healthcare provider immediately. They can make a proper diagnosis and recommend a treatment procedure.

Urethroscopy, physical exam, retrograde urethrogram, and urethra imaging are popular urethra stricture tests you may undergo before being treated for the condition (Urology Care, n.d.).

Stenosis

A person's spinal cord runs through their spinal canal, their vertebrae's tunnel. Stenosis narrows the spinal canal of someone's lower back and strains their muscle nerves or spinal cord. Walking distances become difficult for people with spinal stenosis. They may also feel discomfort in their legs or experience bladder or bowel complication (Johns Hopkins, n.d.).

Osteoarthritis and joint syndromes are common causes of spinal stenosis. Other circumstances that may provoke stenosis include rheumatoid arthritis, previous spinal surgery, spinal tumor or injury, and particular bone infections.

If you have stenosis, you may experience symptoms like chronic leg weakness or numbness, back distress, and cauda equina syndrome (CES), a lumbar region disorder.

The treatment your doctor recommends will depend on your symptoms and diagnosis. Whether you have abnormal reflexes, sensation loss, or body weakness, your healthcare provider will conduct a physical examination to substantiate your condition. Other tests include a lumbar spine X-ray and CT or MRI scan (Johns Hopkins, n.d.).

Hemorrhoids

If your anus or lower rectum has swollen veins, you may have hemorrhoids, but nothing is certain until your healthcare provider runs a proper diagnosis. Approximately 50 percent of older adults (50 years and above) suffer hemorrhoid symptoms (Kahn & Jewell, 2021). Hemorrhoid or pile has two variants – internal and external. While internal hemorrhoids develop within the rectum or anus, external hemorrhoids affect the outside of the anus.

External hemorrhoids are more problematic and common, and often provoke severe irritation, itching, and sitting difficulty, but they are remediable. Hemorrhoid symptoms depend on their variant. Internal hemorrhoid clues include bloody stool and bulged anus, while anus pain, itching, and sitting difficulty may characterize external piles.

Hemorrhoids may disappear without medication, but consult your healthcare provider if you have bloody or black poop. Pile complications are rare, but hemorrhoid patients may suffer skin tags (after symptoms disappear), anemia, swollen veins, infection, and blood clots (Kahn & Jewell, 2021).

If you want to avoid piles, understanding hemorrhoid risk characteristics can help. Potential catalysts include chronic diarrhea or constipation, obesity, anal sexual intercourse, and constant heavy lifting.

Colon Polyps

Colon polyps occur when someone's rectum or large intestine's internal lining reaches abnormal growth. There are sessile (slightly raised) and pedunculated (stalk-supported) polyps. Without proper medical attention, polyps can grow to become cancers.

Thirty percent of those in the 45–50 year age range have polyps (Cleveland Clinic, 2020). Several circumstances, including genes, lifestyle, aging, and diet, can trigger colon polyps. Other catalysts include alcohol misuse, obesity, smoking, and excess processed food consumption.

Colon polyps may not show noticeable symptoms, so healthcare providers often recommend screening, but common signs are rectal bleeding, anemia, iron deficiency, bowel habit alterations, and unusual weight loss. Should you experience these symptoms, consult your healthcare provider for a proper diagnosis. Special procedures for identifying (and remedying) colon polyps include colonoscopy, sigmoidoscopy, CT (computerized tomography) scan, and stool tests. Your doctor will determine the appropriate procedure for you.

Colon Cancer

In 2020, life expectancy in the U.S. dropped by 2.1 years, from 76.3 to 74.2 (Sullivan, 2021). Joining the senior citizens' demographic is a great feat but is also another reason to give gut health close attention to avoid colon cancer. Older adults, according to recent studies, have a higher risk of contracting colon cancer (Mayo Clinic, 2022).

Colon cancer starts as noncancerous clusters (polyps) in the large intestine. Since polyps show no symptoms, healthcare providers suggest screening examinations recognize and eliminate polyps before they become harmful cancerous cells.

Common colon cancer symptoms include unexpected bowel habit alterations, bloody stool, bloating, severe abdominal pain, rectal bleeding, fatigue, and sudden weight loss. Medical experts are investigating colon cancer's general causes, but common risk factors include:

- **Older Age**: If you are 50 years or older, you have a higher risk of colon cancer.
- **Race**: African-Americans suffer colon cancer more than other nationalities.
- **Personal History**: If you've been diagnosed with noncancerous polyps, you have a higher risk of developing colon cancer.
- **Inflammatory Intestinal Disorders**: People with Crohn's disease, ulcerative colitis, and other persistent inflammatory conditions may develop colon cancer.
- **Gene Mutations**: HNPCC (hereditary nonpolyposis colorectal cancer) and FAP (familial adenomatous polyposis), like several inherited syndromes, can trigger colon cancers.
- **Family History**: If you have a family member or blood relative with rectal or colon cancer, you have a higher risk of developing the disease.
- **Smoking and Alcohol**: Heavy smokers and alcohol consumers have a greater risk of colon cancer.

Inflammatory Bowel Disease (IBD)

Approximately three million Americans suffer from IBD, and most victims fall between 15 and 30 years old (Cleveland Clinic, 2021). Whether you're male or female, nobody is immune from inflammatory bowel disease, such as ulcerative colitis, microscopic colitis, and Crohn's disease, IBD's three major types. Anyone who contracts the disease may experience persistent intestinal distress and swelling.

Crohn's disease can provoke discomfort and swelling in the digestive tract. While it often affects the large and small intestines, other GI parts may also be affected. Ulcerative colitis may result in colon and rectum ulcers, while microscopic colitis can induce intestinal inflammation. Common causes of IBD include:

- **Genetics**: If someone in your family has experienced IBD in the past, you may suffer from the ailment.
- **Immune System Response**: If you have IBD, your immune system may react to certain foods, sparking IBD symptoms (Cleveland Clinic, 2021).
- **Environmental Triggers**: Depression, smoking, pills, and stress, like many ecological catalysts, can induce IBD symptoms in individuals

with an IBD family history.

General IBD indications or symptoms include abdominal discomfort, bloating, diarrhea, appetite loss, fatigue, bloody stool, stomach upset, weight loss, and vision problems. IBD patients have a higher risk of contracting colorectal cancer. Other complications such patients may develop include:

- Severe intestinal bulging
- Perforated bowel
- Malnutrition or malabsorption. The small intestine won't provide the body with adequate nutrients
- Bile duct inflammation, cirrhosis, and other liver disorders
- Kidney stone(s)
- Blood clots and red blood cell shortage

Signs of a Super Healthy Gut

As we have learned, several factors, including antibiotics, sleep, stress levels, and food intake, can impact our gut health, but how can we evaluate our own health? Watching for these signs can help:

- **Poop Habit**– If you poop three times daily or weekly, you have a healthy gut. Pooping should also occur during the daytime. Getting up at night to poop may indicate gut problems. Mark Pimentel, gastroenterologist, Associate Professor of Medicine and Executive Director of the Medically Associated Science and Technology (MAST) program at Cedars-Sinai Medical Center, explains that normal poop should occur in the morning after we wake up. Diurnal pattern, as he describes it, makes the colon contract and discard its waste content (Galloway, n.d).
- **Gut Transit Period**– Knowing how long it takes for the food you eat to be digested and move through your gut system is important when examining gut healthiness. The transit time may be about 28 hours, although it varies from person to person (Zoe, 2021).
- **Perfect Poops**– Consistent poop color and shape may suggest that your gut is healthy. If your poop is brown (medium or dark), you have a healthy gut system. If it's yellow, green, red, or black when you didn't eat beetroot or other colored foods, consult your doctor (Zoe, 2021).
- **Pain-free Pooping**– If pooping makes you uncomfortable, go for a gut check. Irritable bowel syndrome, food intolerances, and constipation are common causes of pain when pooping.

- **Stomach Gurgles**– Stomach growling does not always mean you're hungry. It could indicate that you have a healthy gut. It is often experienced after 90 minutes without a meal (Galloway, n.d).
- **Insufficient Gas**– A healthy gut causes us to fart between 10 and 20 times daily, but holding in gas may trigger unfavorable health consequences. Trapped gas may cause bloating.

Practical Steps: Check Your Gut Health

Despite the preponderance of autoimmune disorders and chronic illnesses, concentrating on gut well-being should be a priority for anyone who craves better health. Almost everything about us, including our hormones, immune system, and mental fitness, is attached to our gut. Shifting attention from our health can subject us to many medical conditions.

Checking, not guessing, your gut condition will help you understand the steps you need to take to improve your gut health. For example, if there are any severe health issues to address, you can't know until you undergo proper gut testing. Regular health reviews can keep you on track and also guarantee quick recovery (Unbound Wellness, 2017).

Making modifications without adequate testing may trigger disastrous consequences, and wrong gut protocol or treatment can harm your body system. But a successful gut healing journey is impossible without proper testing. Following these logical steps may help when establishing your gut health:

Visual Inspection: If there's any gut or digestion problem, examining your poop can help. A physical poop analysis will show what's happening to the gut and the foods that your system struggles to digest or absorb. Poop can change each time you visit the toilet because the meal you consume may change your poop habit (Unbound Wellness, 2017). Consider these things when inspecting your poop:

– **Stool Color**: If you have health issues, your stool color can help you identify them. Colors to consider include:

- **Greenish-yellow or Pale**– If you have fat malabsorption or bile duct impediment, you may have a greenish-yellow or pale stool. Bile duct constraint and fat malabsorption are poor digestion problems.

Reaching out to a healthcare provider is crucial when this condition lingers. Your doctor can check your gall bladder. A nutritionist can advise you on what to do to facilitate fat digestion.

- **Red or Black Stool–** Red or black stool may indicate internal bleeding, so reaching out for immediate medical help is critical, unless you have recently consumed beets.
- **Green Stool–** If you ate tons of veggies, you might have a green stool, especially when your system doesn't digest them properly. Improper digestion turns nutrients to waste. So, cooking greens and chatting with a nutritionist on viable strategies to boost digestion may help.
- **Yellow Stool–** If you suffer intestinal inflammation or infection, you may have a yellow stool. Consult your healthcare provider if your stool suddenly turns yellow.

Are you worried about your sinking or floating stool? If your stool contains many nutrients, it sinks quickly. If you aren't digesting fat properly, your stool will float (Unbound Wellness, 2017).

– The Beet Test: If you want to know the time it takes for food to run through your digestive system, conducting a beet test can help. Understanding your transit time (the period food runs through your digestive system) helps determine whether your GI tract is dormant or highly active. While a sluggish digestive system causes constipation, your system may not absorb essential nutrients if it has a swift transit time. Here's how to do the beet test:

- Eat a meal with beets and record the time you ate.
- Wait until the beets pass through and watch for purple or red stool.
- Record your findings. While there's no conventional standard, you should achieve results between 24 and 48 hours. If you record different results after two beet tests, consult your nutritionist or healthcare provider.

– Functional Stool Analysis: A functional stool analysis helps you have a clear view of what's happening to your gut. It entails sending your stool sample to a laboratory for assessment. Findings can have an impressive impact on how one manages their gut health.

Stool examination has different varieties. So, being specific about what you want helps healthcare providers know the appropriate stool test for you. However, a functional stool analysis may capture the following:

- Existence of particular microflora strains
- Enzyme levels
- Specific fungal or bacteria overgrowth
- Leaky gut, fat indigestion, and other nutrient malabsorption

- Parasite infection

If you're interested in having a stool analysis conducted, contacting a functional medicine healthcare provider will help. They can ensure you receive a high-quality stool test.

– **Lactose Breath Test**: If you experience SIBO (small intestinal bacteria overgrowth) or chronic bloating, asking your healthcare provider to conduct a lactose breath test could help you discover what's wrong with your gut system.

For this test, your doctor will ask you to change your diet for one day and drink a lactose (sugar) beverage before they take your breath samples. After screening the samples, they will know whether your small intestine has bacteria overgrowth. Lactose breath test are the most effective diagnosis for suspected SIBO cases (Unbound Wellness, 2017).

Workbook Questions

As you've seen, our gut microbiome can significantly impact our overall well-being, including our moods and happiness level. Studying and answering these questions should improve your understanding of the concepts discussed in this chapter.

- Can you justify why the gut microbiome is tagged as the body's second brain?
- How would you differentiate functional GI disorder from gastrointestinal syndrome?
- What are common risk factors for lactose intolerance?
- How do people know they have a healthy gut?

Eliminating unhealthy practices like drug or alcohol misuse can help your gut microbiome. Should you suffer any persistent symptoms, seek medical attention. The next chapter endeavors to explain the science behind a leaky gut.

4

A SCIENTIFIC APPROACH FOR
FIXING YOUR GUT

Investigations about the gut microbiome continue to generate surprising outcomes. For example, based on one's gut biodiversity, researchers can tell if they are slim or overweight. Also, being the body's second brain, your gut significantly impacts your happiness, morale, and overall mood (Viome Blog, n.d.). Regrettably, our lifestyles (such as staying indoors, taking antibiotics, and living in an urban environment) are weakening our gut microbiome diversity and exposing us to gut permeability, also known as the leaky gut. This chapter will discuss leaky gut and what science tells us about it.

Leaky Gut Hypothesis and Symptoms

Much like Monica in Chapter One, Sonia's body never returned to full health after having a child nine years ago. She had mild depression, fatigue, joint distress, low libido, sleeplessness, and digestive difficulties, but thought that being a busy mom had triggered these symptoms. Based on her healthcare provider's recommendations, she was tested for mononucleosis, thyroid disorders, anemia, and Lyme disease, but again like Monica, all tests came back negative. Her doctor advised her to get more sleep and avoid stress.

When Sonia finally saw a California nutritionist, she was advised to start a food diary and undergo food sensitivity and allergy tests, just as Monica had been. Results showed that Sonia had a leaky gut and was very sensitive to soy, gluten, sugar, dairy, and caffeine, all things she consumed daily. Whether or not you're a mom, if you're experiencing stomach upset, unexplained weight loss, fatigue, or other GI tract disorders, visiting a nutritionist may help. But now you're probably wondering, *what does leaky gut mean?*

The human gut is a complex system responsible for digesting food and absorbing nutrients. The intestinal lining plays a critical role in this process, as it allows for the absorption of water, nutrients, and other compounds from the food we consume. However, in some cases, this permeable lining can become damaged, leading to what has been termed "leaky gut."

A leaky gut occurs when the intestinal lining develops holes or cracks, allowing undigested food particles, toxins, bacteria, and other harmful substances to leak into the bloodstream. When these foreign compounds enter the bloodstream, they can trigger an immune response, leading to food sensitivities and other health issues.

Research has shown that an imbalance of gut bacteria, which we've learned is called dysbiosis, is one of the leading causes of leaky gut. When the balance of beneficial and harmful bacteria in the gut is disrupted, the harmful bacteria can overpower the good bacteria, leading to inflammation and damage to the intestinal lining.

Individuals with persistent gastrointestinal tract ailments, such as Crohn's disease or celiac disease, are more likely to suffer from a leaky gut. However, a leaky gut can also occur in individuals with no preexisting condition, as a result of poor diet, stress, medications, and other lifestyle factors.

Although the leaky gut remains a scientifically unproven hypothesis, researchers say it may cause autism, multiple sclerosis, and other poorly understood ailments (Pisharody, 2015). The surface area covered by the abdomen's intestinal lining is over 4,000 square feet. When functioning properly, it regulates what goes into the bloodstream, but an unhealthy stomach lining has cavities and cracks. Toxins, bugs, and partly digested food particles penetrate the bloodstream via these holes. This circumstance can cause gut flora imbalance and provoke inflammation and other persistent diseases (Campos, 2021).

The human body is a marvel of complexity and intricacy. One aspect that is particularly fascinating is the gut lining. It is interesting to note that the lining of our gut is akin to our external skin, which has been turned inside out. It acts as a barrier that separates the "outside" world from our internal organs. The gut lining plays a vital role in keeping harmful substances out while allowing necessary nutrients to pass through.

The gut lining shields our body from harmful toxins and pathogens that we may ingest along with our food. At the same time, it is also responsible for allowing beneficial substances like carbohydrates, fats, and proteins to flow smoothly through the digestive tract.

It is not uncommon for skin problems, such as psoriasis, acne, and eczema, to be related to issues in the gut. There is an intricate connection between the gut lining and the condition of our external skin. Therefore, it is imperative to keep our gut healthy if we want to maintain healthy skin.

Internal bleeding, which can be a terrifying experience for anyone, occurs when there is bleeding within the gut. The gut lining acts as a safeguard against such internal bleeding.

Leaky gut studies are increasing because researchers believe the medical condition can cause or contribute to conditions like irritable bowel syndrome, asthma, hepatic steatosis, type 2 diabetes, and several disorders. In dealing with gut permeability, investigators often recommend probiotics, dietary shifts, and relevant interventions. Researchers maintain that physiological stressors (like intensive work out and anxiety) and emulsifiers (and other nutritional ingredients) can trigger gut permeability and make toxins infiltrate the circulatory system (Hollander & Kaunitz, 2019).

Who can develop a leaky gut? Whether through food sensitivity or a genetic predisposition, nobody is invulnerable to gut permeability. Your DNA isn't the only culprit; the modern lifestyle can trigger gut inflammation. For example, the regular American diet may precipitate a leaky gut because it has excess saturated fats and sugar but low fiber content. Stress and alcohol abuse can harm gut health as well (Campos, 2021).

Although many healthcare professionals consider LGS (leaky gut syndrome) a non-diagnosable ailment, recent studies showed it could cause celiac disorder, polycystic ovary disease, persistent liver infection, food sensitivities and allergies, and other medical conditions. For example, a 2016 review found that gut microbiota imbalance and intestinal permeability could cause gut inflammation. A 2017 study concluded that a leaky gut could provoke depression, anxiety, and other mental health illnesses (Eske, 2019).

Diagnosing gut permeability is complicated because other health conditions share their signs. However, significant leaky gut symptoms we can all watch for include:

- Continual bloating, diarrhea, or constipation
- Depression, anxiety, confusion, or difficulties with concentration
- Severe joint pain, fatigue, or headache
- Eczema, rashes, acne, or other skin problems

What to Believe: Is Leaky Gut a Real Thing?

Healthcare professionals hadn't wholly understood disease-causing mechanisms when hundreds of years ago some physicians discovered that abdomen imbalance could trigger specific ailments, a condition they called hypochondriasis. The word, derived from ancient Greek, refers to "the soft parts between the ribs and navel" (Campos, 2021).

As science developed and sophisticated microscopic tools (that supported viruses, parasites, and bacteria viewing) evolved, the term changed. Doctors started using hypochondriac to describe chronic, unexplainable medical conditions. What if all major health issues originate from gut imbalance? Can a dysfunctional GI tract provoke the persistent ailments confronting humans today?

While bloating, discomfort, food allergies, and fatigue are common leaky gut symptoms, the condition remains a medical mystery. For example, Donald Kirby, gastroenterologist and Director of the Center for Human Nutrition at the Cleveland Clinic, explains that gut permeability is a relatively gray area because healthcare providers hardly understand the gut microbiome (DerSarkissian, 2022).

If you have developed leaky gut symptoms, but your doctor isn't diagnosing gut permeability, don't criticize them or feel bad because nobody teaches about leaky gut syndrome in medical school. Linda Lee, gastroenterologist and former Clinical Director, Division of Gastroenterology and Hepatology at Johns Hopkins University School of Medicine, said healthcare providers know there's a leaky gut but do not really understand the condition.

Since clinical tests rarely specify leaky gut causes and other illnesses share gut permeability symptoms, many people do not receive the appropriate diagnosis and treatment. Finding a physician who understands your concerns is key when dealing with leaky gut syndrome.

Root Cause of Leaky Gut Syndrome

If an individual suffers from an autoimmune disorder, their healthcare provider may suggest they ditch soy, gluten, and dairy products, but what happens if their condition doesn't improve after they've tried everything they've been told to do? Altering one's diet may help with chronic ailments, but when symptoms don't improve after three months, it's probably time to dig deeper.

Anyone with autoimmune disorders, such as Hashimoto's disease, may experience leaky gut, but intestinal permeability triggers vary from one individual to another. Leaky permeability root causes include:

- **Gluten Sensitivity**: One in five people living with rheumatoid arthritis, Hashimoto's disease, or other autoimmune conditions is gluten-sensitive. Gliadins, a component of gluten, are proteins present in wheat, and can unsettle and weaken the intestinal cells (Wentz, 2021).

Even people without celiac disease may experience sensitivities if they eat foods containing gluten. As gluten escapes into the bloodstream, it can cause gut-related reactions. People who consume gluten regularly have higher risks of developing leaky gut.

- **Food Sensitivities**: Some people are reactive to the proteins in quinoa, corn, rice, and other gluten-free grains. Dr. William Davis, author of *Wheat Belly*, believes that many people are sensitive to difficult-to-digest foods (rice, corn, and quinoa), soy, nuts, seeds, dairy, and eggs. For example, a recent study of over 2,000 Hashimoto patients showed that 58 percent reacted to gluten, 45 to dairy, and 28 to soy (Wentz, 2021).

Food sensitivity symptoms may include palpitations, skin lesions, headaches, fatigue, joint pain, and irritable bowel syndrome. Triggers of food sensitivity are leaky gut, stress, and inflammation.

- **Zinc or Glutamine Depletion**: The human body uses glutamine and zinc to rebuild the impaired intestinal lining. Individuals with low stomach acid may struggle to absorb zinc from proteins, while vegans and people on low animal protein diets may not get the required glutamine their body needs. Red meats, oysters, and other animal products are rich in zinc, while eggs and dairy have sufficient glutamine.

- **Parasites**: Over 30 percent of Americans live with parasites, but the existing detection procedures skip several parasites when one is tested (Wentz, 2021). Parasitic infections such as Giardia, H. pylori, and Blasto are popular leaky gut triggers. Parasites can create holes in the intestinal wall and cause autoimmune disorders and food sensitivities. Worms, protozoa, and amoebas are common parasites affecting gut health, and dealing with them early on can help.

- **SIBO (small intestinal bacteria overgrowth):** Factors like poor diet, low stomach acid, and antibiotic misuse may cause gut bacteria overgrowth and provoke gut permeability. For example, 50 percent of hypothyroidism patients, according to a 2007 review, had SIBO (Wentz, 2021). Acid reflux, bloating, and belching (after consuming veggies and fermented or fibrous foods) could be SIBO symptoms.

- **Fungal Infections:** Recent research has shown that fungus (Candida infection) can trigger food sensitivities and autoimmune disorders. Excess carbohydrate consumption, certain medications, and high stress levels can expose one to Candida infection. Pathogenic yeast may also undermine the intestinal wall and cause intestinal permeability.

The Gut-in-a-Dish Model

Intestinal permeability remains the primary scapegoat for leaky gut syndrome, but recent research suggests it could be more toxic than originally feared. Older people, cancer (or other chronic disease) patients, and individuals with stressful lifestyles often experience leaky gut. Stressors crack abdomen cell walls (or gut lining), prompting leakage of molecules and microbes, an immune response, and chronic inflammatory conditions such as atherosclerosis, cancers, inflammatory bowel disease, and arthritis.

Healthcare providers have no specific treatment for leaky gut, but researchers from the University of California have been utilizing 3D models of patients' intestinal cells to duplicate leaky gut conditions. With this development, clinicians are able to better understand intestinal permeability (including its molecular signals) and how to diagnose, evaluate, and track its advancement and treatments. Gastroenterologist and University of California, San Diego Professor of Medicine and Cellular and Molecular Medicine, Dr. Pradipta Ghosh, led this study and co-authored their findings, which was published in *Life Science Alliance* journal in February of 2020 (Buschman, 2020).

Along with her colleagues, Ghosh discovered a mechanism that could tighten the intestinal lining junctions, which they called the stress-polarity pathway.

They realized the intersections suffered when the pathway became stressed and also learned that metformin (a diabetes medication) could stimulate the pathway to fix the junctions. However, these findings came from Petri-dish-grown cell lines and might not work in humans.

Ghosh and her team changed concentration and developed 3D models using patients' gut organoids. They discovered that humans have rough gut lining with multiple gorges and ridges. Many tiny stem cells lie under each gorge, and the researchers took some stem cells from patient donors and took them to the lab, where they developed. The cells did as they would in a human gut by growing into four distinct cell categories, but swiveled up to form crypts or mini-gut balls. To understand leaky gut circumstances, the researchers exposed the crypts to different bacteria types, and the gut lining junctions fell apart. This discovery showed that the stress-polarity pathway could impact gut junctions.

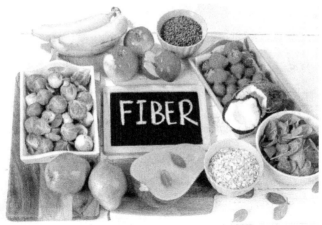

The Importance of FIBER

Fiber is often overlooked when it comes to maintaining gut health. It's like the unsung hero in the story of your body; it's important, but you don't realize *how* important until it's gone. The consequences of not including fiber in your diet can be disastrous!

Without fiber, our bodies become weak and vulnerable to disease and illness, much like a house without a strong foundation is vulnerable to collapse or damage from storms. Fiber acts as a barrier - it feeds the microbiome. In absence of fiber, the bacteria start feeding on 'mucin' which is a protective layer on the gut lining. This disrupts the microbiome where bacteria start to overgrow and inflammation increases. It's like an all-you-can-eat buffet for bad bacteria that can lead to digestive problems, nutrient imbalances, allergies, food sensitivities and a weakened immune system. Studies have identified this as the major reason for leaky gut and other immune system diseases (Usuda et al., 2021).

Now, this is not a one-off event - it is compounding, like a snowball rolling downhill. You start with a small imbalance and this affects your microbiome balance, which leads to more imbalance. This cycle continues until you reach a tipping point where things can no longer be reversed.

If your diet lacks fiber, your gut lining will start to thin out and break down, resulting in leaky gut syndrome and increased intestinal permeability. Increasing your fiber intake is one of the best ways to improve your overall gut health!

The importance of fiber to gut health is so great that the common deficiencies we worry about - vitamin D, protein and calcium - pale in comparison. A diet devoid of fiber leads to an array of nutrient deficiencies along with poor digestive health. Aging, autoimmune and metabolic diseases all have strong links to fiber deficiency. You NEED to focus on getting fiber.

Fiber is an essential nutrient for maintaining a healthy lifestyle. Studies have shown that it provides multiple benefits to our bodies, including repairing the blood-brain barrier, preventing and reversing insulin resistance, and even reversing coronary artery disease. The consumption of fiber-rich foods can also lower the risk of developing type 2 diabetes, heart disease, and obesity.

Unfortunately, despite the known benefits of fiber, studies suggest that only 3 percent of Americans are getting sufficient amounts in their diet. The recommended daily intake of fiber is 25 grams for women and 32 grams for men, yet most people are falling short of this recommendation.

Moreover, research has shown that fiber may have preventive effects against Alzheimer's disease. Studies have found that individuals who consume high levels of fiber are less likely to develop this debilitating condition. It is believed that soluble fiber has a positive effect on the gut microbiome, leading to a reduction in inflammation, which is associated with Alzheimer's.

Incorporating fiber-rich foods such as fruits, vegetables, whole grains, nuts, and legumes into our daily diet is crucial for good health. Consuming enough fiber can improve digestion, lower cholesterol levels, and promote a healthy weight. It is a nutrient that cannot be overlooked, and we must ensure that we are meeting our daily fiber needs.

Now different types of fiber have different effects on our body, because they feed different types of bacteria. For example, resistant starch is broken down and absorbed by the gut bacteria to produce short-chain fatty acids (SCFAs), which are then used by the intestines as energy. SCFAs also act as a barrier to bad bacteria, keeping the microbiome healthy and balanced. The fatty acids also play a vital role in reversing leaky gut and preventing colon cancer.

Natural killer T-cell activators, such as soluble fibers, help with the production of killer T-cells. These cells play a vital role in the immune system by destroying virus-infected and cancerous cells. Fiber can also help reduce inflammation because it keeps bad bacteria from overgrowing and helps maintain a healthy microbiome.

There is a direct connection between our gut microbiome and the strength of our immune system. 70 percent of our immune system lives in our gut through the bacteria and other microorganisms, so a healthy gut will mean a healthy immune system. Improved glycemic control, improved cholesterol levels, and even improved mental health have all been attributed to a high-fiber diet.

Additionally, all the major metabolic disorders can be prevented with adequate fiber intake.

To our bodies, fiber is essentially indigestible; however, the bacteria living in our gut depend on it for sustenance. As they feed, they produce beneficial metabolites, which can help protect and repair the gut lining, promoting better digestive health. Unfortunately, many people fail to consume enough fiber, and as a result, the gut lining deteriorates, leading to a wide range of complications and diseases. This underlines the importance of including fiber-rich foods in one's diet.

Aside from fiber, another important aspect of a healthy diet is the inclusion of polyphenols. Polyphenols are natural antioxidants, typically found in plants such as berries, nuts, and vegetables. They have been found to be beneficial in many ways, including their ability to increase our energy levels. This is because they are known to "uncouple" mitochondria – the energy-generating organelles. This process can help support good metabolic function, reducing oxidative stress and limiting inflammation.

In addition to directly benefiting our bodies, polyphenols also feed our gut bacteria, acting as prebiotics. This promotes healthy microbial growth, helping to enhance digestion and overall health. In light of this, incorporating polyphenol-rich foods, such as dark chocolate, green tea, and red wine into our diet can be a great way to improve our health as well as our energy levels.

So, if you are serious about your gut health and want to make sure your body is well-equipped to fight off any kind of immune system disorder, then fiber should be at the top of your list. Make it a priority in your diet and reap the benefits - better digestive health, stronger immune system and improved overall health!

The Importance of Fermented Foods

Fermented foods have long been a part of human diets worldwide, and while they were a necessity for preserving food in the past, today they are primarily consumed for their potential health benefits. Fermenting food involves allowing it to sit and steep in bacteria, which convert the carbohydrates into organic acids like lactic acid. This conversion process enhances the flavor and texture of the food while also producing probiotics and other beneficial nutrients that can improve digestion and overall health.

Numerous studies have been conducted on the gut microbiome in recent years, highlighting the essential role of microorganisms in maintaining health. A healthy gut microbiome is critical not only for digestive health but also for various other bodily functions, including immune system regulation, metabolism, and even cognitive function. Fermented foods have been shown to contribute to a healthier gut microbiome by introducing beneficial bacteria that can help crowd out harmful bacteria and restore balance to the gut environment.

Some examples of fermented foods include yogurt, kimchi, kefir, miso, sauerkraut, tempeh, and kombucha. These foods are rich in vital nutrients like B vitamins, enzymes, and probiotics that support the digestive process and immune system function. For example, fermented dairy products like kefir and yogurt contain beneficial strains of bacteria that can ease digestive discomfort and promote healthy digestion. Kimchi and sauerkraut are fermented vegetables that are often used as condiments, and they contain prebiotic fibers that feed the beneficial bacteria in our gut. Kombucha is a fermented tea that is rich in antioxidants and probiotics and is a popular health drink for its purported ability to boost energy and improve overall health.

Incorporating fermented foods into your diet is a simple step you can take to improve your gut health and overall well-being. They are easy to prepare, and their unique flavors and textures can add variety and interest to your meals. It's recommended to start slowly and introduce fermented foods in small amounts to avoid digestive discomfort.

Let's Check the Science

Understanding the relationship between eating and feelings is necessary when remedying gut permeability. While excess meal consumption precipitates bloating, a healthy breakfast nourishes and energizes the body. Diarrhea and constipation, like many digestion problems, affect many Americans, and diet remains the primary culprit. If you have chronic intestinal permeability or gut sensitivity, eating these foods may help:

- **Bananas and Leaky Gut**: Whether you choose the smooth-skinned, lustrous, or large varieties, bananas can boost gut health, regulate bowel function, reduce bloating, and lower cholesterol. Banana starch acts as a prebiotic and increases beneficial gut bacteria. Bananas also contain potassium and micronutrients that benefit heart health (Lewin, 2021).

In addition, eating bananas may help alleviate heartburn. For example, since unripe bananas contain leucocyanidin, eating them can improve stomach mucous membranes and counteract stomach acid.

Bananas may also improve mood since the body converts its tryptophan content to serotonin, the feel-good hormone that reduces anxiety, enhances mood, and aids relaxation.

- **Eggs and Leaky Gut**: Eggs aid digestion and prevent digestive problems like ulcerative colitis and constipation, but they could trigger intestinal gas in some individuals because they contain sulfur. Vitamin D in eggs is good for gut health (Lawson, 2018).
- **Apple Cider Vinegar and Gut Health**: With tons of vitamins and polyphenols, apple cider vinegar is an excellent antioxidant source, and consuming it regularly can prevent cellular damage and gut permeability. Its blend of beneficial bacteria can boost a healthy digestive system (MiNDFOOD, 2020). It also contains quercetin and pectin. While quercetin improves gut barrier integrity, pectin regulates gut bacteria and curbs inflammation (Lawson, 2018).
- **Avocado and Leaky Gut**: If you experience leaky gut or digestive difficulties, eating avocado may help, since it contains tons of fiber.

A single avocado has approximately 10 grams of soluble and insoluble fiber. Medical professionals affirm that fiber can curb bloating and constipation (Pingel, 2021).

Insoluble fiber melts stool (and ensures it doesn't become too bulky), while soluble fiber regulates blood sugar and digestion.

- **Coconut Water and Leaky Gut**: Coconut water contains essential nutrients such as potassium, calcium, sodium, and magnesium, and drinking it can curb dehydration and boost heart health, blood volume, and muscle relaxation. Also, cytokinins in coconut water have anti-cancer properties that impede cancer cell growth or development (Levy, 2018).
- **Lemon Water and Leaky Gut**: The fiber and vitamin C in lemons can improve gut health. Vitamin C combats gut inflammation, boosts the immune system, and prevents free radicals from attacking body cells. Its antimicrobial content also regulates gut bacteria (MiNDFOOD, 2020).
- **Ginger and Leaky Gut**: If you suffer from constipation, bloating, or other digestive issues, consuming ginger may help. Ginger can improve digestion, combat inflammation, and relieve migraines, heartburn, and nausea (Mindd Foundation, n.d.).

Its antiparasitic, antifungal, and antibacterial properties make consuming ginger suitable for people with leaky guts. It also aids gastric juice and stomach acid production and facilitates digestion.

- **Fish Oil and Leaky Gut**: Omega-3 and 6, fish oil essential fatty acids, are suitable for brain health and also prevent digestive problems, inflammation, and heart disease. The IAP (intestinal alkaline phosphatase) in fish oil can also prevent gut permeability.

Case Study 1: *Amanda had been living with puzzling gastrointestinal symptoms for months. She experienced frequent bloating, irregular bowel movements, and nausea. Suspecting a food intolerance, she eliminated certain foods from her diet. Unfortunately, that wasn't enough to rid Amanda of her symptoms. In an attempt to find relief, she began drinking lemon water in the morning and incorporating ginger into her meals. While this helped a bit, she was still feeling ill and decided to visit a gastroenterologist and nutritionist for help.*

Amanda underwent detailed food sensitivity/allergy testing as well as other lab tests to determine the root cause of her distress. After reviewing her test results, the nutritionist informed Amanda that she could be suffering from leaky gut syndrome and provided helpful strategies for addressing it. It was recommended that she adopt a diet low in sugar and focus on eating plenty of fiber-rich foods like legumes, fruits, vegetables, nuts, and whole grains - all of which support healthy gut bacteria and boost digestion. Additionally, activities such as yoga and meditation were encouraged to reduce stress levels, which can exacerbate leaky gut issues.

Upon implementing the suggested dietary and lifestyle modifications, Amanda was overjoyed to discover that her well-being had significantly improved. She experienced an immediate decrease in symptoms such as bloating, nausea, and irregular bowel movements, which had previously plagued her daily life. By incorporating a greater quantity of fiber-rich foods into her diet and effectively managing stress using yoga and meditation, Amanda succeeded in healing her leaky gut. As a result, she not only alleviated her immediate discomfort but also secured long-term relief from her digestive issues, paving the way for a healthier and more balanced life.

Workbook Questions

Healthcare professionals believe there's a close connection between what we consume and our overall well-being. While visiting a medical specialist is important when you develop intestinal permeability symptoms, paying attention to what you eat can help you avoid gut-related problems. Answering the following questions will boost your leaky gut understanding and help you maintain a healthy gut bacteria balance.

- What are leaky gut tell-tale root triggers and symptoms?
- If an individual develops gut permeability, what foods should they eat, and why?
- What role does fiber play in relation to intestinal permeability?

Lifestyle plays a key role in combating leaky gut syndrome. Lack of exercise, drug misuse, alcohol abuse, and other unhealthy habits can sabotage gut health. In the next chapter, we will discuss gut health cleansing.

PART II

THE 4-WEEK GUT HEALTH
HOLISTIC NUTRITION PLAN

5

GUT HEALTH WEEK 1: CLEANSING

Feeling nervous, moody, or embarrassed could be gut disorder symptoms. If you suffer unexpected constipation, diarrhea, bloating, food intolerances, or your poop becomes unpredictable, going through gut cleaning procedures may help. Healthcare professionals recommend gut cleansing to patients because they believe it can improve their health and general well-being.

Whether fixing a weakened gut or eliminating food particles that exacerbate or jeopardize gut health, having a gut cleanse can be a valuable step in balancing gut bacteria or accomplishing optimal gut health. The first week of the gut health protocol discussed in this book will help you understand how to cleanse your gut.

Can You Cleanse Your Gut?

Gut or colon cleansing is the comprehensive removal of toxins and waste from the colon, and it's beneficial to health complications like IBM (irregular bowel movement) and constipation. Medical consultants believe gut cleansing can promote healthy weight loss, digestion, energy, and constructive thinking. With water, diet, and maybe some over-the-counter medication, you can do a natural gut cleansing at home (White, 2022).

Why colon cleansing? If the gut malfunctions, food digestion or absorption suffers. While the gut ensures your body receives adequate nutrients, metabolic waste and toxins flow from the circulatory system into your stomach. A healthy gut terminates infection-causing microorganisms and ensures your body absorbs essential nutrients, minerals, and vitamins (PHWC, n.d.). If you're looking for natural colon cleansing ideas for inspiration, the following can help you maintain a healthy gut system:

- **Hydration–** Staying hydrated and drinking lukewarm water can boost digestion. Eating watermelons, celery, lettuce, tomatoes, and fruits with high water content also helps (White, 2022).

- **Saltwater Flush–** If you suffer constipation or poop abnormalities, undergoing a saltwater flush may help (although we still need more scientific evidence to authenticate its potency). Seeking proper medical advice before doing a saltwater flush is highly recommended.

- **High-Fiber Diet–** Seeds, vegetables, nuts, fruits, and grains have healthy fiber amounts. Fiber aids digestion, regulates overactive bowels and constipation, increases helpful bacteria, and eliminates the colon's toxic substances (White, 2022). Eating fiber-rich foods is an effective natural gut cleansing strategy everyone can trust.

- **Stay Active–** Regular workouts can boost detoxification function and gut health. Exercise also reduces the risks of type 2 diabetes, cancer, and heart disorder (PHWC, n.d.).

- **Juices and Smoothies–** Regular consumption of vegetable or fruit juice is good for gut health. In addition to aiding hydration, vitamin C in fruits and vegetables can improve gut health.

- **Herbal Teas–** Aloe vera, slippery elm, and marshmallow root, like other laxative herbs, may ease constipation. Ginger, cayenne pepper, and garlic have sufficient antimicrobial phytochemicals to suppress harmful gut bacteria.

Obtaining a doctor's approval before gut cleansing is advised, especially since colon cleansing has many consequences. Side effects of intense cleansing may include electrolyte imbalances, dizziness, cramping, bowel perforation, dehydration, and nausea. Since these symptoms can trigger digestive trauma or heart failure, discontinue the process if side effects persist (Schaefer, 2018).

How to Do a Saltwater Flush for a Clean Colon

Constipation is not something to be ashamed of, because one out of every five people experiences it. If the digestive condition doesn't change or improve after regular intake of fiber-rich foods, undergoing the saltwater flush may help. Saltwater flush, also called master cleanse or saltwater cleanse, is a GI tract cleaning procedure that boosts bowel movement.

As a popular fasting and master cleanse detox component, people use saltwater flush to treat persistent constipation, cleanse the colon, and detoxify their body system. The process encompasses combining non-iodized salt with warm water and drinking the mixture. Advocates say it eliminates the parasites, toxins, and waste materials in the colon.

Since saltwater flush can stimulate rapid bowel movements, some say it is an effective short-term colon cleansing procedure. Still, no scientific research has confirmed the removal of parasites or toxins, or the effectiveness of body detoxification. While there is plenty of anecdotal proof and online testimonies, chatting with your healthcare provider before undergoing the procedure is essential.

A recent review in the *Journal of Alternative and Contemporary Medicine* found that interchanging specific yoga drills with drinking lukewarm saltwater could boost colon cleansing (McDermott, 2019). What remains ambiguous in this study is whether only drinking the lukewarm saltwater can generate similar results. Understanding the potential risks of a saltwater flush should help you decide whether or not to utilize it. For example, if you haven't eaten breakfast, you may experience nausea, bloating, vomiting, and cramping after drinking saltwater. It may induce sodium overabundance and high blood pressure.

Saltwater flush isn't suitable for everyone. If you have high blood pressure, a heart situation, edema, diabetes, kidney issues, or GI problems (like inflammatory bowel disease or ulcers), avoid this colon cleanse procedure (McDermott, 2019). It should be a pre-breakfast activity because that's when it's most effective. If you're doing it later, ensure you eat nothing for two or three hours beforehand (Axe, 2021).

Here's how to do the saltwater flush:

1. Combine 2 teaspoons of Himalayan or sea salt and 1 liter of warm, distilled water in a cup or glass.

2. Add 1/2 teaspoon lemon juice and shake thoroughly until the salt

dissolves.

3. Drink up within five minutes.
4. Lie on your side and massage your stomach. Switch sides and stroke your belly again.

Staying at home is necessary because saltwater flush will force you to use the bathroom often until your colon is thoroughly cleansed. If possible, take probiotic supplements and eat healthy foods after having a saltwater flush (Axe, 2021).

Delicious Herbal Tea Recipes for Cleaning the Gut

Fitness professionals and health-conscious individuals know the importance of gut cleansing. Detoxifying could be an immediate remedial formula for medical complications. Urbanization and its toxic-laden atmosphere have adverse health impacts on people's lives. While the body does natural detoxification via the liver, urine, sweat, and excretion, the existence of atmospheric toxins and heavy metals continues to threaten human health. Internal detoxification can be quite beneficial, and drinking these herbal tea recipes can help:

- **Detox Haldi Tea**: Many people enjoy this wonder-spice turmeric tea because of its multiple health benefits. Turmeric contains anti-inflammatory components that ease discomfort and ease depression and arthritis symptoms. Its antioxidant properties can also improve skin health and the immune system. If you want a homemade detox haldi tea, here's how to prepare it:

1. Simmer 1 cup of water in a skillet or saucepan.
2. Stir in black pepper, ginger, and turmeric, and simmer for five minutes.
3. Steep and serve.

- **Ginger and Turmeric Tea**: While turmeric contains vital nutrients and anti-inflammatory and antioxidant properties, ginger can soothe bloating and many digestive problems. Drinking tea prepared with ginger and turmeric can strengthen your gut health and overall well-being.
- **Nettle Tea**: The roots, stems, and leaves of heart-shaped nettle plants are boiled to prepare nettle tea. When touched, the plant's tiny hairs often trigger a harsh sensation, but drinking nettle tea is perfectly safe. The polyphenols in nettle tea help the body combat inflammation. Regular nettle tea consumption can energize the

lymphatic system and boost waste excretion via the kidneys. Herbal health practitioners use nettle plants to treat urinary tract infections and other urologic problems.

- **Fennel Tea**: Fennel can improve digestive function, alleviate constipation, and aid colon cleansing. If you're drinking fennel tea, don't exceed one cup daily because you need to analyze how your bowels react to it. Fennel tea can boost antioxidant activities and prevent the liver and kidneys from oxidative stress.
- **Tulsi Tea**: Drinking this natural detox tea can improve metabolism and purify your gut system. It also supports healthy weight loss.
- **Detox Ajwain Tea**: Carom or Ajwain seeds can relieve tension, indigestion, and constipation and also promote healthy weight loss. Follow these steps to make your flavorful and healthful Ajwain tea:

1. Mix some ajwain seeds with 1 cup of water in a pan.
2. Simmer the mix for 2 or 3 minutes.
3. Add honey to taste, and serve.

- **Lemon Tea**: The vitamin C in lemon tea can boost the immune system and combat infections. Combine lemon tea with plain water, turmeric, and black pepper, and you will have a flavorful, refreshing drink. Its superb detoxing qualities make it a must-have for everyone.
- **Peppermint Tea**: Vitamin C in peppermint can boost the immune system and protect the body against virus and bacteria infection, and its manganese content helps neutralize free radicals. Peppermint tea can also aid digestion and remove mucus that impedes air passage.
- **Dandelion Tea**: Urination is an outstanding means of removing toxins from the body, and dandelion root facilitates peeing. The plant aids kidney and liver cleansing and also contains immune-enhancing antioxidants.
- **Detox Cinnamon Tea**: Chefs use dalchini or cinnamon to flavor curries, soups, and stews because it's delicious and has several health benefits. Cinnamon's anti-diabetic properties can strengthen the body's insulin response. Its antioxidants also secure the body against free radicals. Here's how to make homemade cinnamon tea:

1. Mix some cardamom pods, ginger, cinnamon sticks, and 1 cup of water in a pan.
2. Boil the mixture for 2 or 3 minutes, seep and serve.

- **Green Tea**: Drinking green tea can improve gut health and facilitate a natural colon flush. Green tea contains immune-enhancing properties, and EGCG (epigallocatechin-3-gallate), its potent antioxidant, can prevent liver-related ailments, including liver cancer. Green tea also has L-theanine, the glutathione-producing amino acid. Being an antioxidant, L-theanine combats free radicals.

- **Plain Ginger Tea:** Drinking this tea may help when you develop a sore throat or flu. Ginger contains body-cleansing properties, and it is a detoxifying tea you can trust anytime. Adding a pinch of cardamom to your ginger tea can improve its taste.

- **Milk Thistle:** You may wonder whether this recipe contains dairy but its milky flavor comes from the thistle plant. Milk thistle supplements can curtail inflammation and liver damage and stimulate cell repair. Herbal health practitioners have used milk thistle to treat liver-related issues for hundreds of years, but little evidence supports its potency.

Check out your local grocery store for any of the herbal teas listed above.

Case Study 2: *Alice had been suffering from digestive issues for years. Her stomach was often in knots and she was constantly bloated, sluggish, and experiencing heartburn. She decided to take matters into her own hands and try a colon cleanse over a three-day weekend. The first few days provided only slight relief, but Alice was determined to achieve the results she wanted.*

She found a longer plan that included detox teas and an entire meal plan to follow. She cut out all unnecessary sugars, caffeine, dairy, and alcohol that she had been consuming regularly before the cleanse. During the week-long plan, Alice felt an immense transformation in her body, as if it was being reborn. Within just a few days of following the new diet and drinking herbal teas, her bloating subsided and her stomach no longer burned with acid reflux.

Alice was amazed at how quickly her gut health had improved from the changes to her diet. Not only did it make her feel less sluggish physically, but mentally she was at ease knowing her digestion was functioning correctly once again. This newfound sense of well-being motivated Alice to continue adhering to this lifestyle change in order to maintain optimal gut health in the future.

7-day Healthy Lifestyle Changes for Cleansing the Gut

Clean digestion and nutrient absorption, including efficient toxins processing by the liver, are crucial to excellent health. If you want to strengthen your immune health or rejuvenate your body, embracing a gut cleanse procedure can help. You can experience a comfortable colon wash if you prepare your body for lifestyle changes. Avoid processed foods, refined sugars, coffee, cigarettes, alcohol, and saturated fats five days before a gut cleansing program, because they can increase the toxins in your body.

Consuming fiber-rich foods like vegetables and fruits is an important step to maintaining a clean colon. Drinking eight (or more) glasses of filtered water daily can facilitate body detoxification. Avoid stressful situations, because they can endanger gut health. Paying attention to what you eat, drink, and think or feel also helps. Observing these 7-day healthy lifestyle changes for gut cleansing should keep you active and strengthen your overall well-being.

Day 1– Sipping lemon-spiced herbal tea is rejuvenating and a beautiful way to start a detox diet plan. Halve a lemon and squeeze it into your herbal tea or warm water and enjoy! Engaging in light workouts like swimming, a bike ride, brisk walk, or yoga can bolster your fitness.

- **Breakfast**: Raw vegetable juice. Options include spinach, carrots, celery, wheatgrass, beetroot, coriander, kale, and mint. Blending the juice with one tablespoon of chia seeds can boost its fiber content.
- **Lunch**: Lightly simmered or fresh vegetables. Healthy options are onions, pumpkins, broccoli, beetroot, mushrooms, ginger, cabbage, spinach, garlic, carrots, mustard leaves, capsicum, and fenugreek leaves.
- **Dinner**: Vegetable stew. Here's how to prepare it:
  - Sauté garlic, onions, and veggies in a saucepan.
  - Add sea salt to taste and 2 cups of water.
  - Cook for at least 10 minutes (or until the vegetables become edible).
- **Snacks**: Drink herbal tea and tons of water. Eat apricots, guava, apple, strawberries, plums, oranges, pears, and other low-GI fruits.

Day 2– Mix lemon with herbal tea (or warm water), drink up the mixture, and do your swimming, bike ride, walking, or yoga routine.

- **Breakfast**: Mix 1 tablespoon of blended chia seeds with your favorite raw vegetable juice and drink.
- **Lunch**: Quinoa with baby spinach salad and lightly boiled veggies.
- **Dinner**: Stir-fry garlic and lemon juice, broccoli drizzled with olive oil and capsicum with vegetable stew.
- **Snacks**: Select from the Day 1 snack list.

Day 3– Repeat your early morning lemon-herbal tea (or warm water) routine and light exercise.

- **Breakfast:** Add sliced fruits, walnuts, and almonds to 3/4 cup of yogurt. Garnish it with fresh honey and enjoy. Sip herb or green tea.
- **Lunch:** Veggie and lentil stew. Here's how to prepare it:
  o Combine small ginger and garlic clove pieces, 1 cup veggies, 1/2 cup yellow moong dal, and 2 cups water in a saucepan.
  o Drizzle olive oil and stir in salt according to your taste.
  o Cook for at least 15 minutes (or until veggies and dal soften).
  o Coat with parsley and enjoy.
- **Dinner:** Fresh carrot and papaya salad. Follow these steps to prepare it:
  o Combine 1/2 fresh papaya, 1 finely chopped carrot, 2 cups lettuce, and 1 tablespoon vinegar in a container.
  o Drizzle fresh lemon juice and 1 tablespoon of olive oil, and serve.
  o Snacks: Select any of the Day 1 snacks.

Day 4– Start the day with your lemon-herbal tea and light activity habit.

- **Breakfast:** Coconut-banana smoothie. Here's how to make it:
  o Combine 1 tablespoon of chia seeds and coconut oil, 100 grams of natural coconut milk, and 1 banana in a blender.
  o Blend for 3 minutes or until you have a smooth-textured smoothie.
- **Lunch:** Amaranth (or quinoa) with vegetable stew.
- **Dinner:** Veggie and lentil stew.
- **Snacks:** Choose from the Day 1 variety.

Day 5– Begin with the lemon-herbal tea mixture and workout routine.

- **Breakfast:** 1 tablespoon of blended chia seeds with raw veggie juice.
- **Lunch:** Boil fresh herbs with veggies. Sprinkle in mashed pumpkin seeds and olive oil. Combine the mixture with almonds and 1/2 cup rice.
- **Dinner:** Rocket leaf salad. Follow these steps to prepare it:
  o Mix thinly chopped red capsicum strips, onion and mushroom slices, and fresh rocket leaves.
  o Drizzle with sunflower seeds, fresh herbs, lemon, and olive oil, and serve.
- **Snacks:** Any of the Day 1 snacks would be fine.

Day 6– Drink your regular lemon and herbal tea drink and do your usual yoga, brisk walk, or swimming session.

- **Breakfast**: Combine dried prunes, flaked almonds, apricots, 2 tablespoons ground flaxseed, soaked and filtered apples and peaches in a container. Enjoy it with plain yogurt.
- **Lunch**: Amaranth and 1/2 cup rice with veggie and lentil soup.
- **Dinner**: Fresh carrot and papaya salad.
- **Snacks**: Choose from the Day 1 snack list.

Day 7– Repeat the early morning herbal tea beverage and workout.

- **Breakfast**: Coconut-banana smoothie.
- **Lunch**: Veggie and lentil soup garnished with greens, raisins, almonds, and lemon juice.
- **Dinner**: Mashed potato, 1/2 cup rice, and green salad grilled with mushrooms.
- **Snacks**: Choose a snack from the Day 1 snack list.

If you followed the 7-day gut cleanse diet above, congratulations! You should feel fresh, strong, and rejuvenated. Continue to eat healthy meals to maintain your gut health and overall well-being. Starting your day with a warm lemon water drink helps stimulate digestion.

Foods you shouldn't consume during the 7-day gut cleanse include mints, chewing gum, artificial sweeteners, and refined sugars. You should also avoid caffeine, alcohol, butter, ice cream, sour cream, cheese, yogurt, milk, and other dairy products.

Artificial sweeteners are known to cause a wide range of health issues, from mild digestive disturbances to more chronic and serious conditions such as obesity, type 2 diabetes, and various metabolic disorders. This can lead to impaired digestion and nutrient absorption, as well as increased risks of developing food sensitivities, allergies, depression and anxiety. Artificial sweeteners have also been linked to changes in appetite and cravings for sugary foods.

These adverse effects on health can be even worse if one regularly consumes large amounts of artificial sweetener over a long period of time. Even small doses ingested over time can contribute to systemic inflammation that can lead to other health issues. Given these alarming facts, it's clear why it's important to opt out of consuming any kind of artificial sweetener during the 7-day gut cleanse diet.

7-day Gut Cleanse Meal Plan

If you don't want to call off the procedure halfway through, make sure you've readied all your provisions before starting a detox or gut cleanse meal plan. These include:

- Herbal teas and purified water
- Coconut milk, almond, and other dairy-free milk products
- Greens and seasonal fruits
- Miso, sauerkraut, kefir, kimchi, and other fermented foods
- Coconut aminos, apple cider vinegar, and tamari
- Nuts, salmon, coconut oil, seeds, olive oil, and other healthy fats
- Tempeh and tofu (for vegans) or free-range, GMO-free chicken
- Sprouts
- Psyllium husk (for additional fiber)
- Turmeric, garlic, ginger, and other spices or herbs

The body can run a natural detoxification process, but the foods mentioned above can facilitate colon cleansing and your diet. In other words, one's diet may have a negative or positive impact on how the liver and kidneys remove toxins from the body system. A natural colon cleanse becomes complicated when one continues to consume poor food. These diets can help stimulate natural gut cleansing:

- **High-Fiber Foods**: Consuming fiber-rich foods (or fiber G supplement) in the 7-day gut cleanse period helps. It curbs constipation, calms overactive bowels, enhances colon health, and increases the beneficial gut bacteria. Foods like vegetables, fruits, nuts, and seeds have a healthy amount of fiber.
- **Herbal Tea**: Regular herbal tea consumption can boost digestive health. You can have two or three cups of herbal tea daily. However, if you're consuming laxative herbal tea, have it only once a day. Common laxative herbs include aloe vera, slippery elm, and psyllium. Although laxative herbal teas may improve constipation symptoms, excess consumption can hurt your overall well-being. Healthy herbal teas are garlic, cayenne pepper, and ginger. They aid in elimination of harmful gut bacteria.
- **Gut Cleanse Foods**: Kale, broccoli, avocado, turnips, and cabbage are common natural detox foods. Cauliflower, spinach, tomato, and carrot can improve kidney, liver, and gut health. These foods help consolidate the digestive system and also house vital antioxidants and

anti-inflammatory properties. For example, vitamin A in carrots curbs liver infections, while tomatoes prevent liver damage. Spinach also reduces liver fat. Adding foods with enough water also helps when implementing a 7-day gut cleanse meal plan. Foods within this category include tomatoes, watermelon, celery, cucumber, and lettuce. Health benefits offered by the gut cleanse diet include enhanced heart health, improved mood, healthy weight loss, and better-quality sleep. Use these meal ideas to design your own 7-day gut cleanse diet plan.

Early Morning Routine: A warm lemon water drink can energize and activate your digestive system. Drinking water before meal consumption can improve digestion. If your gut cleanse meal plan requires any supplements, this is the time to take them.

Morning Options: A sugar-free breakfast is excellent for gut health. Breakfast food and drink suggestions include:

Chia Pudding– Eat chia pudding one hour after the early morning routine. Here's how to make this delicacy:

- Mix 1 cup of almond and coconut milk with 1/2 cup chia seeds in a container.
- Refrigerate it for a few hours.

Peanut butter-sweetened avocado toast– Whole-grain bread is a good choice, but gluten-allergic individuals can choose gluten-free varieties. Avocados contain vital minerals, vitamins, and healthy fats.

Spicy Green Waffle– If you want to nourish your digestive enzymes and gut system, eating this delicious recipe can help. Green waffles contain tons of probiotics, and you may garnish them with strawberries, bananas, or honey.

Overnight Oats– The aroma of this versatile and delectable recipe is quite enticing, and you can make it at home.

- Blend 2 tablespoons of Greek yogurt with 1/2 cup of tossed porridge oats in a container.
- Keep the mixture in the refrigerator for 2 hours.
- Add maple syrup or your favorite fruits.

Lunch Options: Eat sugar-free meals when cleansing your gut. Healthy lunch food options for stomach cleanse include:

Lemon-Garlic Baked Salmon– Omega-3 fatty acids can improve gut health, and salmon has enough of it. Garlic contains prebiotics, and lemon has immune-strengthening vitamin C.

- Line the baking sheet in a 400-degree preheated oven and lay your fish on it.
- Sprinkle olive oil, minced garlic, and lemon juice on the fish.
- Bake for 10 minutes (or until the fish turns crispy).

Veggie Burrito Bowl– Here's a 100 percent plant-based gut cleanse treat you just can't resist. It's made with medicinal herbs like cilantro, avocado, arugula, and fiber-rich cauliflower.

Marinara Sauce with Zucchini Spaghetti and Chicken Meatball– Gut cleansing shouldn't prevent you from enjoying a fancy dish.

Let's make the meatballs first:

- Mix 2 cloves garlic, 1 pound chicken (ground), 2 eggs, and 1 tablespoon of nutritional yeast and flaxseed in a container.
- Add pepper and salt to taste, and blend thoroughly.
- Form the mixture into balls and bake at 350 degrees in a preheated oven for 20 or 25 minutes.

Now to make the marinara sauce:

- Simmer 2 tablespoons olive oil in a skillet or saucepan.
- Blend 1 teaspoon oregano, 28 ounces peeled tomatoes, 2 diced garlic cloves, and 1 onion in a container.
- Pour the tomato mixture into the saucepan and cook for 45 minutes.

Let's prepare the zucchini noodles:

- Cut your favorite veggie into tiny slices, lengthwise.
- Heat olive oil in a skillet, add the zucchini noodles and simmer for 2 or 3 minutes.

Blend the zucchini pasta, marinara sauce, and meatballs, and serve.

Snack Options: Minimize your snack consumption during the 7-day gut cleanse period. However, healthy snack choices include an apple, 1/2 cup blackberries, 10 almonds, hummus and pepper slices, and a Clementine.

Dinner Options: Choosing any of these meal selections should boost your gut health:

Turkey Meatball Soup and Kale– Spice this healthy delicacy with turmeric, and you'll surely want to have it another day.

Miso Vinaigrette with Green Salad– This delicious light dinner is made with healthy and gut-friendly greens like arugula, kale, broccoli, and spinach. Feel free to add some chia seeds, almonds, sprouts, flax seeds, and cashew nuts.

Mix 1 tablespoon apple cider vinegar, 1/2 teaspoon mashed ginger, 2 tablespoons of orange juice, 3 tablespoons of olive oil, and 1 tablespoon of water in a bowl to make the salad dressing.

Lettuce Wraps (Thai-Style)– Preparing this healthy gut-friendly delicacy is very simple; follow these steps:

- Mix yellow onion, celery, veggies, chopped carrots, 1/4 cup tamari, diced ginger and garlic, some honey, and 2 tablespoons apple cider vinegar in a saucepan.
- Add 2 tablespoons of water and simmer for 12 minutes (or until the veggies become tender).

Exercise can also strengthen gut health, but choose yoga or light workouts during your 7-day cleanse. The cleanse diet may be observed anytime, but not without the guidance of a healthcare provider.

Workbook Questions

Gut cleansing is vital to everyone's well-being, and making healthy lifestyle changes helps. Answering these questions will improve your understanding of this chapter.

- How would you describe colon cleansing, and how does it benefit humans?
- What are common gut cleanse ideas discussed in this chapter?
- Can you describe how to do the saltwater flush?
- Can you identify three or four delicious herbal tea recipes for colon cleansing?

Unexpected food intolerances, constipation, bloating, diarrhea, and even anxiousness and moodiness could be indications you need a colon cleanse, but seek medical advice before modifying your diet or undergoing the gut cleansing process. In the next chapter, you will learn more about gut healing and rejuvenation strategies.

6

GUT HEALTH WEEK 2: HEALING AND REJUVENATION PROTOCOLS

Nutrition, or what an individual consumes, is critical to their gut health. And, since the gut is the starting point for so many diseases, prioritizing gut well-being is vital. The second week is about what to do to heal and rejuvenate a leaky gut using 100 percent natural means.

Fasting and Gut Health

The tiny living organisms in our abdomen have an incredible impact on our body's balance. A sudden diet alteration (what we consume, food size, and when we eat our meals) can unsettle the gut's natural harmony. Many people understand this much, but learning how gut microbes derive their potency is equally valuable in discovering the impacts of fasting on the gut microbiome.

Animal researchers conducting investigations on the consequences to gut health of intermittent fasting proved that altering eating habits could improve immune health and act as a promising therapy for diabetes. Many of these studies were carried out on mice, so clinical trials with humans are still required to either uphold or dismiss these theories.

Certain fasts, according to recent studies, may improve blood pressure, regulate blood glucose, and prevent diabetes, heart disorder, high cholesterol, and other chronic medical conditions. Still, the influence of the gut microbiome in all these remains unclear. Krista Varady, Professor of Nutrition at University of Illinois, believes that available surveys did not show how (and to what extent) intermittent fasting helps one's appetite, sleep, and microbiome (Putka, 2021).

While some human studies investigated fasting effects on the gut microbiome, people's reactions to fasting differ. Scientists must determine what happens to the gut when we fast before anyone can claim or argue that fasting triggers the alteration of the gut microbiome. Researchers have shown that what and when one eats may shift their gut composition or balance.

While one survey found that Akkermansia (a beneficial bacteria genus) increased in mice that fasted for 16 or 20 hours, another study showed that individuals who practiced the 16:8 fasting method recorded no substantial variation in their microbiome composition or balance. The 16:8 fasting procedure calls for fasting for 16 hours and feeding for eight hours.

A 2021 study on how intermittent fasting and the microbiome impact weight management found that short dietary modifications do not affect the gut. Maintaining a dietary shift or long fast for a few weeks or months, however, may impact gut bacteria, boost heart health, and regulate blood pressure. For example, scientists examined the effects of five days of fasting on individuals on a Mediterranean diet in a 2021 clinical trial. Results showed that participants' blood pressure was regulated, and their gut microbiota experienced considerable alterations.

While fasting may have had notable improvements in microbiome-linked health problems in many animal studies, what helped mice may not yield positive outcomes in humans. One study, for example, found that intermittent fasting reduced cognitive impairment and triggered microbiome changes in mice. In another study, researchers concluded that intermittent fasting could prevent vision damage, retinopathy, and diabetes in mice (Putka, 2021). Several studies have also shown that fasting and/or various forms of time-restricted eating extends lifespan and longevity. For reference, a study published in the journal *Nature Communications* in 2015 found that a 40 percent reduction in food intake extended lifespan in mice and delayed age-related diseases.

Whether one experiments with time-restricted feeding or a weekly fasting schedule, timing is essential. Researchers maintain both procedures stimulate healthy weight loss, boost metabolic function, and ease cancer and diabetes risks. But pregnant women, breastfeeding mothers, and individuals with eating disorders should avoid fasting (Schwartz, 2020).

Here are fasting types you can practice to increase microbiome diversity and strengthen your gut health if you choose:

- **Time-restricted eating** plan requires fasting during particular hours or periods of the day. The eating schedule includes 20:4, 16:8, and 14:10. Sticking to the 16:8 eating plan, for example, means you fast for 16 hours and eat for 8 hours (Vetter, 2022).
- **5:2 fasting** schedule means you maintain your regular food for five days and consume fewer calories in the remaining two days (of the week). Calorie consumption for the two days should be between 500 and 800 calories.
- **Alternate-day** fasting implies rotating the usual eating and fasting days. For example, if you eat on Monday, you can fast on Tuesday, eat on Wednesday, and fast on Thursday.

How to Fast to Heal the Gut

Joe, a gut-health consultant and friend, who himself suffered gut-related health complications in his early 20s, told me that fasting is the quickest means to rejuvenate digestive disorders. His ten-year gut-healing journey motivated him to implement several metabolic and microbiome studies. To improve gut health, Joe said, people should rethink what, how, and when they eat.

While eating puts one in an inflammation (anabolic) growth, fasting puts one in a healing and repair (catabolic) state. Balancing the anabolic and catabolic conditions can benefit gut health. If you suffer certain health complications because your body needs to undergo the catabolic phase to facilitate cellular rehabilitation or healing, changing your diet won't yield desired outcomes. Living anabolic can only aggravate your general health issues.

Fasting for an extended period can balance the microbiome, enhance digestion, and remedy the leaky gut. If you suffer from an inflammatory disorder, malfunctioning metabolism, obesity, poor sleep, or other health complications, healing may come if you engage in intermittent fasting. For example, skipping food considerably reduces immune system apprehension, resets the microbiome, heals the digestive system's lining, and improves symbiotic microorganism multiplicity (Burns, 2019).

Following a fiber-rich or nutrient-dense dinner with a one or two-day fast is a potent gut healing procedure to remedy common wellness disorders and health complications. A well-functioning digestive system and healthy microbiome can regularize bathroom visits, improve body metabolism, aid healthy weight loss, provide substantial energy and boost restful and deep sleep.

Fasting also helps promote mental well-being by stimulating the microbiome to produce neurotransmitters that boost proper cognitive functioning. In other words, fasting can be an antidote for anxiety, depression, and other mental health disorders.

Changing eating schedules or incorporating fasting into your everyday life poses fewer risks than abandoning microbiome health. If your anabolism and catabolism balance becomes compromised, staying fit becomes impossible.

Here are the strategies you should consider when using intermittent fasting to improve your gut health:

- **Remedy Gut Issues First**: Visiting an experienced GI tract healthcare provider may help if you experience dysbiosis or other gut-related health problems. Intermittent fasting can improve your gut-healing efforts and well-being (Pedre, 2022).

- **Evaluate Food Allergies**: If you're sensitive to dairy, soy, gluten, or other foods but eat them anyway, your gut health and fasting efforts will suffer. Avoid foods that unsettle your stomach throughout the fasting period.

- **Eat Fermented and Gut-Friendly Foods**: Eating more kimchi, kombucha, kefir, sauerkraut, and fermented vegetables during the fasting period helps increase beneficial gut bacteria.

- **Blend Keto with Fasting**: Low-carb, high-fat, and moderate-protein diets during fasting can boost microbiome health, and that's what the ketogenic diet offers. Fiber-rich carbs, raw scallions, and prebiotic-dense veggies are the major keto diet components.

Maintaining a healthy gut isn't limited to diet. Poor sleep, stress, and exercise deficiency can undermine your fasting efforts. For example, one study found that regular exercise could positively impact the intestinal microbiota (Pedre, 2022).

Why Use a Leaky Gut Diet for Healing?

From skin rashes or aches to autoimmune diseases, many people believe that major chronic health issues emanate from leaky gut syndrome. Although there's no medical term known as leaky gut, the phrase is attributed to heightened intestinal permeability. Gut-disease connections remain controversial, but researchers contend that gut permeability may trigger celiac disorder, type 1 diabetes, and several persistent autoimmune complications (McAuliffe, 2021).

2016 research found immediate connections between inflammation, gut bacteria concentrations, and intestinal permeability, and a 2018 study concluded that a low gut bacteria biodiversity could provoke inflammation and a leaky gut (Eske, 2019). Diet can impact these conditions. In other words, proper nutrition can improve gut bacteria diversity and help one avoid obesity, inflammatory bowel disorder, and many adverse health conditions. Whatever food an individual is incorporating into their eating schedule, consuming more probiotic and prebiotic foods like sourdough bread, fruits, vegetables, grains, nuts, and seeds can stimulate beneficial gut bacteria growth.

Knowing the food to eat or avoid is critical when remedying intestinal permeability or improving gut health, and this justifies diet as a healing procedure. For example, a well-prepared and nutrient-packed carnivore diet can eliminate the body's toxic substances and inflammatory markers. It also facilitates healing and ensures the body gets sufficient nutrients to thrive.

Here's the point. If your cells aren't receiving adequate nutrients and your gut suffers inflammation, the nutrient supply canal will cut off, and medical complications will likely follow. This explains why gut-health specialists incorporate low-carb and high-fat diets in the treatment of inflammatory conditions. Feeding patients' cells with vital nutrients and eliminating their toxicity pressure can dramatically reduce their inflammatory symptoms.

Meat from animal organs can strengthen gut health because it contains essential nutrients, including water-soluble and fat-soluble vitamins. Excluding vitamin A from your diet for one or two weeks can hurt gut bacteria, undermine your intestinal barrier, and provoke inflammatory bowel disorder. Eating organ meats can help reverse these health issues. For example, 3 1/2 ounces of beef liver has approximately 5,000 micrograms of vitamin A. Salmon roe, pastured lard, and other carnivore foods are rich in vitamin D (McAuliffe, 2021).

Amino acids also promote gut well-being. The glutamine nutrient in beef and eggs can prevent gut permeability, and you shouldn't skip bone broth because its collagen helps repair the bruised intestinal lining.

What to Eat and Avoid on the Leaky Gut Diet Plan

Over 15 percent of Americans suffer from chronic gut sensitivity and digestive issues like constipation and diarrhea (Brennan, 2021). There's a connection between what someone eats and how they feel. While your body gets sufficient energy from a healthy breakfast, you may experience bloating if you overeat. Like low-fiber diets, certain food ingredients can unsettle the digestive system and also increase harmful gut bacteria. Intestinal permeability has also been attributed to excess saturated fat intake.

Consuming probiotic foods at breakfast is an effective way to improve gut health (Foster, 2020). Nourishing gut-friendly breakfast treats include:

- **Overnight Oats**: Mix oats with Greek yogurt to make the meal a creamy texture, and top it with 1 cup of milk to double or triple the food's probiotic health benefits.
- **Probiotic Breakfast Bowls**: Gut-friendly sustenances like scallions, avocado, tangy kraut, and Greek yogurt make up this delicious, protein-packed recipe.
- **Raspberry Ginger Smoothie**: Greek yogurt is a significant ingredient in this nutritious smoothie, but you may substitute yogurt with milk kefir or cottage cheese.
- **Nuts, Maple Syrup, and Yogurt with Potato**: Flavored with Greek yogurt or cottage cheese, sweet potato breakfast can be super nourishing and refreshing.

There is no current recommended medication for leaky gut, but proper nutrition can help you deal with it. Healthy food options to consider when establishing a leaky gut diet plan are:

- **Vegetables**– Gut-friendly veggies include zucchini, beetroot, kale, broccoli, mushrooms, Brussels sprouts, and ginger. Others are cabbage, spinach, arugula, Swiss chard, and carrots.
- **Tubers and Roots**– Turnips, potatoes, squash, yams, carrots, and sweet potatoes are healthy choices.
- **Fermented Veggies**– You can go for miso, kimchi, tempeh, or sauerkraut.
- **Fruit**– Papaya, coconut, passionfruit, grapes, limes, bananas, and mandarin are all good for gut health. Other healthy fruit options are lemons, blueberries, oranges, raspberries, pineapple, and kiwi.
- **Sprouted Seeds**– Sunflower seeds, flax seeds, and chia seeds can improve gut health.
- **Beverages**– Healthy choices include kombucha, bone broth, nut milk, teas, water, and coconut milk.

- **Nuts**– Eat almonds, peanuts, raw nuts, and nut milk to protect your gut and prevent intestinal permeability.
- **Gluten-Free Grains**– Healthy choices include brown and white rice, sorghum, teff, and buckwheat.
- **Healthy Fats**– Choose avocado, olive oil, or avocado oil.
- **Fish**– Omega-3-rich fish like herring, tuna, or salmon help maintain a healthy gut.
- **Cultured Dairy Products**– Traditional buttermilk, Greek yogurt, and kefir can stimulate beneficial bacteria production.
- **Eggs and Meats**– Eating eggs, chicken lean cuts, turkey, lamb, or beef may remedy a leaky gut.
- **Filtered Water** – Consider getting a charcoal filter to ensure you are drinking quality water.

Planning a leaky gut diet isn't just about specifying which foods to consume; knowing what to avoid is equally important to maintaining a healthy GI tract. Eliminate these foods from your eating schedule because they can hurt gut bacteria:

- **Wheat-Based Products**: Couscous bread, wheat flour, cereals, and pasta may unsettle your gut and trigger bloating, constipation, and other digestive problems.
- **Gluten-containing Grains**: Avoid oats, barley, seitan, bulgur, and rye if you have food allergies.
- **Beverages**: Sugary drinks, carbonated beverages, and alcohol can cause digestive issues.
- **Processed Meats**: Hot dogs, cold cuts, bacon, and deli meats are bad for gut health.
- **Artificial Sweeteners**: Saccharin, sucralose, and aspartame, like other artificial sweeteners, can hurt microbiome balance.
- **Baked Foods**: Pizza, cakes, pastries, muffins, pies, and cookies aren't appropriate options for people who value gut health and overall well-being.
- **Junk Food**: Avoid candy, fast foods, sugary cereals, and muesli bars if you want improved gut health.
- **Processed Foods:** As a rule of thumb, you should be eating organic foods instead of highly processed foods whenever possible.

1 Week Fasting Plan with Breaking Meals to Rejuvenate the Gut and Improve Health

Gut health is more about giving your body what it requires, creating a unique, beneficial microbiome, not just consuming fermented foods. Practicing this one-week fasting plan should help improve your gut diversity, curb digestive disorders, and maintain your overall well-being.

One week of doing a one-day on, one-day off fasting and non-fasting schedule can yield many positive outcomes. One reason this fasting procedure is beneficial is that it flushes out the toxic bacteria in your gut more quickly than many gut-healing protocols.

If you want to boost gut diversity, adopting a well-coordinated fasting schedule (like the one you are about to learn here) can help. Fasting helps your body to adjust where and when it needs to. People who omit fasting from their gut diet do so because they don't know that fasting is one of the best ways to rejuvenate the gut.

The last meal before a fast has a more profound effect on the gut microbiome, since you will probably eat a couple of hours after breaking your fast. Eating meals that feed a different bunch of bacteria can stimulate gut diversity. Rotating gut-friendly meals when fasting helps feed the microbiome for an extended period. While the non-fasting days help build up the gut, you may experience bloating during these days.

Cinnamon helps improve gut health, so start each morning with a cinnamon drink. Mix cinnamon with two tablespoons of water and enjoy. Do not drink coffee during your fasting days. While this doesn't mean that coffee is bad for the gut, its acid sometimes discomforts the GI tract. Green tea is advised since it helps restore damaged gut villi.

Fast for 20 hours (or as long as you comfortably can) if you want to derive the maximum health benefits. Probiotics are good but don't take them with food, take them 30 minutes before food. Taking probiotics after digestion starts kills lots of gut microbes, and that's not what you want because it exposes you to several digestive disorders. Have bone broth 30 minutes before you break your fast, and if you like, you can take your probiotics and bone broth together.

Avoid saturated fat, fructose, and glucose when breaking your fast (even one week afterwards). Consuming these substances can negatively affect the gut and also induce intestinal permeability. Break your fast with lean protein, fish, vitamin D, and omega-3-dense foods. Eating low-fat foods is also helpful, but don't exceed 6 ounces of protein and 15 grams of fat when breaking your fast. Consuming more omega-3 fat is good for gut health since omega-3 fatty acids stimulate the gut response the body wants.

Feel free to eat a large meal 60 minutes after breaking your fast. A chickpea and artichoke salad is a good choice. Give your body what it needs to adjust its microbiome when establishing a gut-fast diet plan. It makes the gut flexible and creates more diversity—no further consumption after the large meal until the following sunrise.

The next morning is your non-fasting day. Start the day with the cinnamon drink and follow meals planned for the 7-day Healthy Lifestyle Changes for Cleansing the Gut in the last chapter.

Case study 3: *Jackson had been struggling with his health for some time. He was overweight, hypertensive, and had GERD. After hearing of the potential benefits from intermittent fasting, he decided to give it a shot. He began by fasting for 12 hours each day and gradually increased up to the 16:8 ratio. He incorporated daily morning walks and a window of 9am-5pm that he would adhere to when eating. To start his day, Jackson would have a hearty breakfast after his morning walk and snack throughout the day on almonds and raw vegetables. For dinner, Jackson opted for a variety of fish dishes paired with additional servings of fresh vegetables.*

Thanks to his commitment to the 16:8 fasting routine, coupled with healthy dietary choices and regular exercise, Jackson saw tremendous improvement in his health. His weight decreased substantially as did his blood pressure. Additionally, thanks to changes in his diet and lifestyle habits, Jackson's symptoms of GERD were significantly reduced.

Workbook Questions

With a well-coordinated fasting schedule, managing gut health and remedying digestive disorders has become relatively simple. Since fasting isn't right for everyone, though, consulting your healthcare provider is strongly advised before adjusting your diet, especially if you have diabetes or any chronic health conditions. Answering these questions will help ground your understanding of this chapter.

- How does fasting improve gut health or curb intestinal permeability?
- What fasting categories can one practice to consolidate gut health and boost microbiome diversity?
- How would you describe an effective gut-friendly fasting procedure,

and what crucial strategies should one consider when using fasting to remedy gut disorders?

- What foods should one include or eliminate from a leaky gut diet plan?

Incorporating fasting into nutrition is one natural but effective way to heal or rejuvenate a leaky gut. In the next chapter, we will learn everything there is to learn about eating right.

7

GUT HEALTH WEEK 3:
EATING RIGHT

While the potassium in avocado is double that of a banana, asparagus contains healthy nutrients like zinc, vitamins A, C, and E. Broccoli has a large amount of calcium. The role of nutrition in ensuring and maintaining gut health is discussed in Week 3, along with practical food plans that you can use during this week.

Understanding Probiotics

The gut is home to many bacteria, but some can induce infection (Gunnars, 2020). An average person, according to recent studies, has between 39 and 300 trillion bacteria in their body system. A healthy bacteria blend has several health benefits, such as an enhanced immune system, healthier skin, improved digestion, decreased disease risks, and healthy weight loss. Eating probiotics helps increase the beneficial living organisms (or bacteria) in your body.

Probiotics are healthy bacteria and yeasts inhabiting the body system. An average individual lives with both beneficial and toxic bacteria. The harmful bacteria can cause you to contract an infection after altering your system balance, but the helpful bacteria can eliminate the toxic ones. Consuming probiotic supplements helps enrich the good bacteria and combat diseases (Cleveland Clinic, 2020).

Our microbiome is unique to each of us. Even identical twins have different microbial cells. Probiotic microbes have many features. For example, apart from providing multiple health benefits to the body system and being safe for consumption, probiotics can survive in the intestine after being ingested. Probiotics' primary function is safeguarding the body against toxic bacteria and keeping it healthy.

Good bacteria also strengthen the immune system, supports digestion, creates vitamins, and deters the harmful bacteria consumed from penetrating the bloodstream. But you don't have to consume probiotic supplements before these things can happen. Eating a fiber-rich and well-balanced diet provides your body with abundant beneficial bacteria it needs to stay healthy.

Increasing your probiotic use may help if you have medical conditions like constipation, IBD (inflammatory bowel disease), diarrhea, IBS (irritable bowel syndrome), urinary tract infections, lactose intolerance, and yeast infections (Cleveland Clinic, 2020). If you have diabetes or any chronic conditions, talk to your doctor before altering your diet.

Probiotic-rich foods to multiply the body's healthy bacteria or improve gut health include sourdough bread, buttermilk, kombucha, kimchi, and fermented sauerkraut. Others are kefir, Greek yogurt, tempeh, and cottage cheese.

Probiotics are different from prebiotics, which are mainly fibers and carbs. While probiotics multiply the gut-beneficial living organisms, prebiotics feed them. Symbiotic products contain both probiotics and prebiotics.

Prebiotics

Vegetables. Fruits. Whole Grain. Beans. The food we eat nourishes more than our body system. Microbiomes (the multi-trillion beneficial gut bacteria, also called probiotics, in our body) also benefit from our food. These bacteria require prebiotics (energy-producing nutrients) to flourish. Regular prebiotic consumption, according to studies, can improve probiotics' health. Read on to understand prebiotics and how they impact our well-being.

Probiotics evolve naturally but eating fermented foods, or taking probiotic supplements can make them increase in number. These bacteria consume prebiotics – the nutrients we can't digest or absorb. Prebiotics have multiple health benefits. For example, while particular prebiotics curb gut inflammation and salmonella (food poisoning that causes bacteria) infections, eating fruits and vegetables regularly may prevent colorectal cancers (Wahowiak, 2022).

Prebiotics support healthy microbiomes. They are the nutrients that strengthen the microbiome. Gut bacteria ferment prebiotics to produce short-chain fatty acids, which energize colonocytes and the colon lining cells. Prebiotics also promote beneficial microbes' growth (Kubala, 2022). A compound may be categorized as a prebiotic if it:

- suppresses digestive enzymes (or stomach acid) and does not get absorbed via the GI tract.

- ferments in the intestinal microbes.

- facilitates intestinal bacteria activity or growth to promote health.

Asparagus, tomatoes, chia seeds, dandelion greens, garlic, and Jerusalem artichoke have abundant prebiotics. Other prebiotic food sources include onions and leeks, bananas, seaweed, oats, chicory, beans, wheat, and rye. Adding prebiotic supplements to your diet may help ease gut-related conditions, including high blood sugar (Kubala, 2022).

Prebiotic supplements are readily available as OTC (over-the-counter) drugs in many U.S. supermarkets and stores, and heeding the following tips can help you select a quality product:

- Choose prebiotic supplements with branded ingredients and explore the independent testing types the product has undergone to evaluate its efficacy.

- Choose products with GMP (Good Manufacturing Practices) or USP (United States Pharmacopeia Convention) label certification seal.

Does consuming prebiotics offer the body system any significant health benefits? Prebiotic diets help develop beneficial bacteria and promote digestion. Short-chain fatty acids (prebiotic fermentation by-products) support metabolic and gut health. Prebiotics improve immune function and regulate blood sugar. Other health benefits of eating prebiotics include:

- **Improves Gut-related Conditions**: If you suffer constipation or IBS (irritable bowel syndrome), taking prebiotics may help, since they trigger beneficial bacteria growth. A 2020 study found that inulin (a prebiotic) may reduce IBS and constipation symptoms (Kubala, 2022).

Taking prebiotics may enhance stool frequency, consistency, and intestine transit velocity (the time food requires to travel through the GI tract).

- **Enhances Metabolic Health**: Eating a prebiotic-rich diet and taking prebiotic supplements can regulate cholesterol, blood sugar, and triglyceride levels. For example, one 2019 review found that a particular prebiotic could control insulin and blood sugar levels (Kubala, 2022).
- **Curtails Inflammation Markers**: Prebiotics curb inflammation by strengthening the intestinal lining walls and inhibiting proinflammatory molecule activities.
- **Reduces Body Fat**: Symbiotics (combining probiotics with prebiotics), according to a 2021 study, may trigger healthy weight loss (Kubala, 2022).

Healthful Foods Naturally Containing Probiotics and Prebiotics

Gut bacteria imbalance remains a major infection trigger. Feeding the probiotics with prebiotics helps the gut create the essential short-chain fatty acids that colon cells need to thrive. Metabolic health improves when these nutrients get into the bloodstream. Healthy probiotic and prebiotic food options include:

- **Seaweed** is a versatile probiotic-multiplying marine algae plant that can be used in smoothies, soups, sushi rolls, salads, and other nourishing recipes. The prebiotic-rich food contains ample antioxidants, vitamins, minerals, and immune-enhancing polysaccharides. Seaweed's fiber is mainly soluble, and the polysaccharides in seaweed can boost SCFA (short-chain fatty acid) production. SCFA nourishes the gut lining and enhances gut well-being.

- **Chicory root** is a dandelion flowering plant with a coffee-like flavor when cooked, and it contains a healthy amount of probiotics and prebiotics. Inulin (a prebiotic fiber) makes up 68 percent of chicory root fiber content. Chicory root inulin helps ease constipation, indigestion, and bowel disorder. It also raises the level of the the protein regulating blood sugar levels, and contains enough antioxidants to defend the liver against oxidative trauma (Semeco, 2021).

- **Dandelion greens,** which contain lots of inulin fiber, may be eaten raw or cooked. While one cup of the plant has 1.92 grams of fiber, its inulin fiber improves immune health, increases probiotics, and reduces constipation. Dandelion greens have anticancer, antioxidant, and anti-inflammatory effects on the body. Replacing salad greens with this fiber-rich plant comes with many health benefits.

- **Barley** contains beta-glucan, the prebiotic fiber that boosts probiotics growth, lowers LDL (bad) cholesterol, decreases cardiovascular disease risks, and lowers blood glucose levels. One recent study with mice found that beta-glucan improved mices' appetite, insulin sensitivity, and metabolism (Semeco, 2021). Barley also has abundant selenium, a compound that stimulates thyroid functions and improves immune health.

- **Jerusalem artichoke** looks like a sunflower and has a reasonable amount of dietary inulin fiber. Its inulin compound can improve colon health and digestion. Adding vegetables to the diet may help inhibit metabolic infections, lower cholesterol, and bolster the immune system. The Jerusalem artichoke also has thiamin. Eating this vegetable can help prevent abnormal muscle function and fatigue.

- **Wheat Bran** is pure prebiotics and contains a fiber that boosts beneficial gut bacteria. Wheat bran may also reduce cramping, bloating, abdominal pain, and digestive problems.

- **Asparagus** is a nutritious vegetable and a vital prebiotic source. The flavorful vegetable contains inulin-soluble fiber, which helps boost digestive health and regulate the body's insulin and glucose levels, and also feeds the gut's good bacteria. Asparagus also offers anticancer and anti-inflammatory health benefits.

- **Garlic** is an antioxidant and anti-inflammatory compound source, and offers many health benefits. The tasty prebiotic herb aids growth of a gut-beneficial microorganism and eliminates toxic bacteria. Garlic has anti-tumor properties and regulates blood sugar levels. Eating garlic may help prevent asthma and reduce cardiovascular disease risks as well. (Semeco, 2021).

- **Jicama root** contains loads of prebiotic fiber inulin and vitamin C. Several studies with animals found that consuming jicama root helped improve insulin sensitivity, strengthen digestive health, regulate blood sugar levels, and bolster the immune system (Semeco, 2021).

- **Onions** contain inulin, FOS (fructooligosaccharides), and flavonoid quercetin. FOS strengthens the immune system, aids fat digestion, and improves gut flora, while flavonoid quercetin protects the body against cancer. Onions contain antibiotic properties that enhance the cardiovascular system and also fuel the probiotics.

- **Burdock root** has dietary fiber, FOS, inulin, and phenolic compounds. Eating this root vegetable enhances the growth of probiotics in the gut and helps boost the immune system.

- **Leeks**, onions, and garlic all belong to the same family and provide similar health benefits. Leeks contain inulin fiber, vitamin K, and many other vital minerals. Consuming leeks aids fat digestion, improves gut health, and stimulates blood clotting.

- **Konjac root**, also called elephant yam, is a tuber-like potato. For centuries, Asians have used konjac root as food, medicine, or a dietary supplement. Tuber flour has over 70 percent glucomannan fiber, a dense dietary fiber that boosts probiotics production, relieves constipation, decreases blood cholesterol, and stimulates healthy weight loss.

- **Bananas** are rich in fiber, minerals, and vitamins. They also have some inulin content. The resistant starch in unripe bananas has prebiotic impacts on the microbiome. One banana has about 105 calories, 422 mg potassium, and 3 grams of soluble fiber (Semeco, 2021). Eating bananas helps feed probiotics and eliminate harmful bacteria.

- **Flax seeds** expand healthy gut bacteria, stimulate bowel movements, and reduce the dietary fat digested or absorbed. Flax seeds have phenolic antioxidants and anticancer properties, and consuming them helps control blood glucose levels.

- **Whole oats** offer prebiotic benefits, and they have good resistant starch and beta-glucan fiber amounts. This supports probiotics (healthy bacteria) growth, lessens LDL (bad) cholesterol, improves blood glucose control, and decreases cancer risks (Semeco, 2021). Eating whole oats also helps regulate appetite and digestion.

- **Apples** are a nourishing fruit. They contain loads of pectin, a soluble fiber with prebiotic benefits. Pectin in apples, according to a 2016 study, could decrease inflammation, enhance healthy weight loss, promote probiotics, and eliminate harmful bacteria (Semeco, 2021).

Eating apples also helps boost heart health, curtail pulmonary disorders, and lower asthma risks.

- **Cocoa beans** make smoothies, oatmeal, yogurt, and many recipes healthy and tasty. Crush the beans, remove the coca butter, sprinkle the powder over your recipe, and enjoy. Cocoa contains anti-inflammatory and antioxidant flavonols and compounds that boost probiotics' growth and reduce harmful bacteria.

How to Use Prebiotics and Probiotics for Gut Health

While eating probiotic-rich foods or taking probiotic supplements promotes the growth of beneficial microbes, feeding good bacteria with prebiotics can help them reproduce and colonize the microbiota. We cannot digest or absorb the fibers in our food, but the helpful gut bacteria feed on them, and that's why we often call fibers prebiotics. For example, as we just learned, inulin fiber is found in tomatoes, chicory, asparagus, onion, Jerusalem artichokes, whole grains, bananas, and many other plants.

Prebiotic fibers remain in the intestine after being ingested. Probiotics (the good bacteria) will ferment the fibers and convert them into energy they will use to reproduce and generate good bacteria colonies. Regular prebiotic intake is advised, since abrupt alterations in fibrous diet may trigger abdominal discomfort, bloating, and many other digestive disorders (Kleinfeld, n.d.).

Probiotics and prebiotics foods or supplements may be taken together. Ingesting both can strengthen gut health. While probiotic supplements rejuvenate healthy gut microbes, prebiotic supplements nourish them.

Thankfully, some probiotic supplements contain prebiotics as well, to ensure the probiotics receive adequate nourishment when they hit the large intestine. Prebiotics may be taken separately, of course, and some experts suggest having time intervals between the two supplements can help prevent over-fermentation, a situation that could trigger bloating, gas, and other digestive issues.

Blending probiotics with prebiotics produces these benefits:

- It supports sound bacteria reproduction and eliminates harmful bacteria.
- It enhances probiotic bacteria survival, helps them colonize the intestines, and improves gut health.
- It strengthens the gut microbiota and helps breed beneficial anaerobic bacteria.

Role of Vegetables

Vegetables remain a staple food worldwide, and plant parts we all eat include seeds, fruits, roots, and leaves. Health experts recommend daily consumption of vegetables, since they are low in calories and high in nutrients. Recent studies show that alternating vegetable diets can boost health.

Vegetables have immune-enhancing antioxidants and essential minerals and vitamins. For example, vitamin A in carrots is good for eye health. Other benefits derived from vegetables include:

- **Enhances Digestion**: The dietary fiber in vegetables facilitates digestion and simplifies mineral and vitamin absorption, ensuring the body's system receives an adequate energy supply (WebMD, 2020).

- **Regulates Blood Pressure**: Kale, chard, and spinach, like many leafy greens, have high potassium content. By helping the kidneys to eliminate sodium, potassium regulates blood pressure.

- **Reduces Cancer Risks**: Cancer is responsible for 16 percent of deaths worldwide, but cancer prevention remains the principal treatment, and consuming vegetables can help lessen cancer risks (Ülger, Songur, Çırak & Çakıroğlu, 2018). For example, while the antioxidants in leafy green vegetables safeguard body cells against oxidative damage, their minerals, phytochemicals, and vitamins prevent gastrointestinal cancers.

- **Lessens Heart Disease Risk**: Vitamin K in leafy vegetables can prevent calcium from accumulating in the arteries, which can cause arterial damage and heart-related complications.

- **Controls Diabetes**: Just as their high fiber content aids optimal digestion, vegetables' low glycemic index ensures your blood sugar level doesn't surge after a meal. Daily consumption of three-to-five servings of cauliflower, broccoli, carrots, or other non-starchy vegetables is recommended for diabetic patients, according to the American Diabetes Association (WebMD, 2020).

- **Provides Healthy Nutrients**: Vegetables contain the vital nutrients the body requires to thrive. For example, they contain folate and vitamin B. While vitamin B boosts red blood cell production, folate reduces cancer risks. Other vital minerals provided by vegetables include selenium, magnesium, phosphorus, copper, and zinc.

The nutrient derived depends on the vegetable type and size eaten, of course—

for example, the calories in celery stalk and pea range from 6.5 to 67. The USDA recommends that adults eat one, two, or three cups of vegetables on a daily basis (WebMD, 2020).

Grocery stores have different vegetable varieties, where one may purchase conventionally cultivated or organic blends. Experts suggest regular consumption of other vegetables to maximize their health benefits. Vegetables may be boiled, stir-fried, or roasted before being eaten. If you want to integrate vegetables into your diet but don't know how, here are some tips that may help:

- Combine kale, Brussels sprouts, and cabbage to make a salad.
- Cook zucchini, onions, and peppers together to make a vegetable kabob dinner.
- Mix basil, tomatoes, parmesan cheese, and olive oil and roast in the oven.
- Mix cherry tomatoes, sweet peas, lettuce, and peppers to prepare a fresh garden salad.
- Fry chicken and vegetables with olive oil in a skillet to make a tasty stir-fry.
- Top a toasted cheese sandwich with mushrooms, asparagus, and pepper to create a delicious vegetable melt.

Role of Legumes and Beans

Peanuts, soybeans, green beans, lentils, peas, and lotus, like other edible legumes, contain healthy nutrients like folate, riboflavin, thiamin, and vitamin C. Legumes also have healthy amounts of chromium, copper, zinc, magnesium, iron, potassium, phosphorus, and selenium (Maphosa & Jideani, 2017).

These micronutrients provide many health benefits to the body. For example, while copper improves iron metabolism and enzyme activities, calcium bolsters the bone. Chromium and zinc support lipid and carb metabolism, while iron assists hemoglobin synthesis. Other health benefits of legumes and beans include:

- **Improves Heart Health**: Eating more legumes can reduce heart disease risks. Heart disease's major contributing factors, according to research studies, remain high levels of homocysteine and LDL (bad) cholesterol, but the folate in legumes helps regulate them. Healthcare providers often recommend a soluble-fiber, low-fat, and vitamin B-dense diet for patients with high cardiovascular disease risks because it helps reduce symptoms. Many studies have linked regular bean consumption with reduced LDL cholesterol, including other heart disease markers. One study even reported a 38 percent reduction in nonfatal heart attack symptoms among patients who ate one cup of boiled beans daily. Other studies recorded substantial decreases in blood cholesterol levels of participants who consumed canned beans daily.

- **Manages Diabetes:** Eating different legume varieties helps prevent diabetes and regulate blood glucose levels. Beans contain complex carbs (dietary fiber) that take time to digest. Since eating beans makes someone feel full, it helps control insulin and blood sugar levels after consumption. Legume fiber also curbs metabolic syndrome risks (including diabetes and glucose disorder health issues). One recent study found that regular beans intake could help moderate blood glucose, decrease systolic blood pressure, and reduce risk of coronary heart disorder.

- **Reduces Cancer Risks:** Beans contain cancer-preventing bioactive compounds. Their anticancer effects improve when eaten with vegetables, fruits, and other antioxidant-rich diets. In some animal studies, researchers found that bean intake could reduce risks of prostate, breast, kidney, colorectal, and stomach cancers in humans. For example, the dietary fiber in legumes may help lessen colorectal cancer risks. One study that investigated the effects of dietary fiber on the development of colon polyps found that more fiber intake from boiled peas and beans could hinder polyps' duplication (NDSU, n.d.).

- **Promotes Healthy Weight Loss and Reduces Obesity Risks:** Regular beans consumption has been attributed to reduced waist circumference, decreased body weight, and lessened systolic blood pressure. One Brazilian study linked a conventional rice-and-beans diet to a lower BMI (body mass index).

- **Regulates Blood Sugar:** The resistant starch in legumes helps control blood sugar levels. Beans have a high amount of potassium, fiber, and magnesium. These nutrients help normalize or manage blood pressure (Baranda, 2018).

Role of Fruits

Apples. Oranges. Strawberries. Bananas. If you want to enhance your overall well-being or avoid contracting infections, regular fruit consumption can help.

Fruits contain tons of fiber, minerals, and vitamins, including flavonoids and other immune-boosting antioxidants. Eating high-fruit diets can help you avoid medical conditions like diabetes, cancer, heart disorder, and inflammation (Sissons, 2019). Tangible health benefits of eating fruits include:

- **Curbs Disease**: Eating fruit helps lower heart disease risks, according to a 2013 review. A 2003 Harvard Public Health study also found that eating whole fruits could help regulate blood pressure and control type 2 diabetes (CHF, n.d.).
- **Promotes Bone Health**: Fruits can improve muscle and bone health. For example, eating dried plums may protect against osteoporosis. Tomatoes, avocados, and cranberries can also strengthen bone health. Regular watermelon, figs, bananas, grapefruit, and strawberry consumption is advised because they contain magnesium – the mineral that facilitates calcium absorption.
- **Combats Free Radicals**: Free radicals are unstable molecules that can induce severe health complications like damage to healthy cells and cancer. Eating fruits (especially ripe ones) provides your body with the required antioxidants to combat free radicals, keep you healthy, and boost your gut health.
- **Supports Brainpower**: Berries, like many other fruits, are brain boosters. Eating blueberries, strawberries, and blackberries, as well as other berry fruits, may improve memory loss and other age-related problems (CHF, n.d.).
- **Improves Digestive Health**: The water, fiber, and antioxidant contents in fruits can keep your digestive system healthy. For example, papaya contains papain, an enzyme that boosts digestion and prevents the growth of specific cancerous cells. Bromelain in pineapple also stimulates digestion and reduces inflammation. Other digestion-friendly fruits are strawberries, bananas, and apples.

Role of Foods Rich in Polyphenols

Polyphenols, a classification of compounds in herbs, vegetables, tea, and other plant foods, are antioxidants that help the body neutralize the harmful activities of free radicals. You may have noticed that polyphenol-rich foods have become more popular lately, and this is the reason. It's challenging to stay healthy or avoid significant health issues like cancer, diabetes, and heart disorders without consuming apples, vegetables, red wine, chocolates, and other polyphenol foods (Rodder, 2021). Polyphenols exist in three primary forms – flavonoids, phenolic acids, and polyphenolic amides (Petre, 2019).

- **Flavonoids** exist in foods like red cabbage, onions, apples, and dark chocolate.
- **Phenolic acids** are found in whole grains, vegetables, and seeds.
- **Polyphenolic amides** are in oats and chili peppers.

Other known polyphenols are present in berries, turmeric, and red wine.

Consuming polyphenols comes with these health benefits:

- **Regulates Blood Sugar Levels**: Recent studies show that observing a polyphenol-rich diet helps control blood sugar levels and improves insulin sensitivity. For example, one study found that eating polyphenol-rich foods could lessen the risk of contracting diabetes by 57 percent (Petre, 2019).
- **Lowers Risk of Heart Disease**: The antioxidant properties of polyphenols can help ease severe inflammation, a significant risk factor of heart disease. Polyphenols also help regulate blood pressure and decrease LDL cholesterol levels.
- **Deters Blood Clots**: If you want to reduce your risk of blood clot, eating polyphenol-rich foods may help. Blood clots occur when the bloodstream's platelets clump, a process healthcare professionals call platelet aggregation. Abnormal platelet aggregation can trigger clots, often leading to pulmonary embolism, stroke, deep vein thrombosis, and many other negative health issues. Many animal studies suggest polyphenols could curtail the platelet aggregation procedure.
- **Prevents Cancer**: Antioxidant and anti-inflammatory properties in polyphenol-rich foods may hinder the growth of cancer cells.
- **Promotes Digestion**: Polyphenols help stimulate digestion by enhancing the development of probiotics, the beneficial gut bacteria, and combating toxic bacteria. For example, polyphenol-rich tea aids beneficial gut bacteria growth while green tea polyphenols combat Salmonella, E Coli, and other harmful bacteria (Petre, 2019).
- **Improves Brain Function**: Grape juice is rich in polyphenols, and drinking it may strengthen memory and ability to focus in older adults. While cocoa flavanols may enhance attention and memory, many studies found that consuming Ginkgo biloba (a plant extract

rich in polyphenol) could boost brain activity (Petre, 2019).

Apart from berries, dark chocolate, red wine, and tea, here are other polyphenol-rich foods you might consider to improve your health:

- Fruits like apricots, grapes, pears, pomegranates, and lemons.
- Vegetables like broccoli, spinach, artichokes, carrots, shallots, onions, and lettuce.
- Legumes like white beans, tofu, soy yogurt, tempeh, and soybean sprouts.
- Nuts and seeds like hazelnuts, almonds, walnuts, flax seeds, and chestnuts.
- Grains like whole wheat, rye, and oats.
- Herbs and spices like cumin, star anise, lemon verbena, dried peppermint, curry powder, cinnamon, cloves, and celery seed.

Role of Whole Grains

Many people enjoy eating whole grains because they contain loads of nutrients. For example, while whole grain fiber-rich bran contains abundant antioxidants, iron, zinc, and magnesium, it is also rich in phytochemicals, healthy fat, antioxidants, and Vitamins B and E. The endosperm part of whole grain is home to essential minerals, including carbohydrates and protein. Eating whole grains offers the body system the following health benefits:

- **Reduces Risk of Heart Disease:** According to a recent study, eating 28 grams of whole grains three times daily may help curb heart-related health issues (Jennings, 2019).
- **Curbs Obesity:** Fiber-rich foods prevent overeating because we tend to feel full after eating a high-fiber meal. This explains why nutritionists recommend such foods for healthy weight loss. Whole grain foods have high fiber content.
- **Curtails Severe Inflammation:** Inflammation triggers many persistent infections, but regular whole grain consumption helps ease inflammatory symptoms. For example, one study reported a significant decrease in inflammatory markers in individuals with unhealthy diets immediately after consuming wheat products (Jennings, 2019).
- **Boosts Digestion:** If you suffer from digestive problems, eating whole grains can help because they contain loads of fiber. Apart from

preventing constipation, full-grain fiber serves as a prebiotic and helps feed the healthy stomach bacteria.

- **Decreases Risk of Stroke**: An evaluation of six surveys involving about 250,000 people showed that regular whole grain consumption could reduce stroke risk by 14 percent (Jennings, 2019). Vitamin K, fiber, and antioxidants in whole grains may help prevent stroke.

- **Hinders Type 2 Diabetes**: Whole grain foods with high fiber content help prevent unhealthy weight gain, a key risk factor in diabetes. They also enhance insulin sensitivity and regulate blood sugar levels.

Role of Fermented Foods

Greek yogurt, sourdough bread, kimchi, and sauerkraut, like other fermented foods, taste good and contain loads of beneficial bacteria. Eating these healthy foods can help boost microbiome diversity. The health benefits of eating fermented foods include:

- **Stimulate Digestion and Bowel Regularity**: While yogurt promotes digestion, kefir enhances stool frequency and consistency. Recent studies found that eating sourdough bread resulted in less bloating and abdominal pain than non-fermented bread (Kresser, 2020).

- **Support Bone Health**: Fermented milk products contain essential bone-friendly nutrients like calcium, protein, vitamins D and K2, and phosphorus. For example, eating kefir promotes positive bone turnover.

- **Improve Gut Microbiome**: While kefir helps strengthen helpful gut bacteria, yogurt boosts intestinal Lactobacilli. Tempeh stimulates good bacteria and immunoglobulin A, the intestinal immune reaction trigger. And chocolate supplies prebiotic fibers (Kresser, 2020).

- **Antimicrobial Properties**: Antibacterial and antifungal components of fermented foods help combat harmful bacteria.

Workbook Questions

Eating right is crucial to preventing gut-related health complications or for healing digestive disorders. Answering these questions will help refine your knowledge of this chapter.

- What are the similarities and differences between probiotics and prebiotics?

- Can you identify eight or ten healthy food sources of probiotics and prebiotics?
- How can one use probiotics and prebiotics to improve gut health?
- What are the health benefits of eating vegetables and polyphenol-rich foods?

There is no substitute for eating right when it comes to enhancing gut health and overall well-being. In the next chapter, you will see how to merge exercise with nutrition to boost your gut health.

8

GUT HEALTH WEEK 4: EXERCISE AND MOVEMENT FOR GUT HEALTH

If you want to improve your gut microbiome composition, regular exercise can help. Like prebiotics, exercise helps strengthen the millions of beneficial microbes in your stomach. One recent University of Illinois study found that a mere six weeks of activity could positively impact the microbiome. Fourteen overweight and 18 lean adults took part in the study, in which researchers tested their gut microbiomes and placed them on a six-week, 30 to 60 minutes cardiovascular exercise session, with three sessions daily.

When evaluating the gut microbiomes of the participants after the program, the researchers discovered noticeable alterations – while certain microbes surged, others decreased. For example, many participants had increased gut microbes that boost short-chain fatty acid production. These acids help curb heart disorders, type 2 diabetes, and inflammatory conditions (Pratt, 2018).

Week 4 encourages you to merge your nutrition efforts with exercises that help improve gut health.

The Role of Exercise in Gut Health

Exercise supports our general well-being in diverse ways. For example, it pushes more oxygen into our brain and bloodstream, improving blood flow. Regular exercise also helps strengthen and multiply the beneficial gut bacteria (Chai, 2022).

There's a symbiotic relationship between our body system and many bacteria colonizing our gut. As these microbes stimulate metabolism, our body also supports their growth. For example, the microbiome generates the fatty acids, vitamins, and amino acids the body requires for mood regulation, absorption, and immune functioning. Jacob Allen, Assistant Professor, Department of Kinesiology and Community Health at the University of Illinois, says regular exercise can stimulate the process and help beneficial bacteria thrive.

In a 2018 study, Dr. Allen and his team studied the impacts of six weeks of exercise on gut health. Thirty-two adults took part, and they were divided into two factions – obese and normal weight. The researchers assigned six weeks of supervised training (like brisk walking and spin class) to both groups. Each routine lasted between 30 and 60 minutes, up to three times daily (but there was no alteration to eating patterns or diet).

The researchers collected and analyzed fecal and blood samples from participants after they'd completed the six-week course and found that they had higher short-chain fatty acid levels compared to what they'd had before the procedure (Chai, 2022).

A 2017 PLoS (Public Library of Science) study had similar findings. Forty women within the 18 to 40 age range participated in a 7-day study. Participants were halved, and while one group had three hours of exercise daily, the other group did an hour and a half. The gut microbiota composition of the three-hour activity group improved more than the second group. They also had more beneficial bacteria.

Another study found that regular exercise can boost butyrate production. Butyrate fatty acid helps reduce inflammation and repair leaky gut, preventing insulin resistance and IBD (inflammatory bowel disease). Exercise-provoked microbiota changes can enhance metabolic function and curb obesity. In one review, women who engaged in three hours of brisk walking, swimming, and other light workouts per week saw an increase in their probiotics, as opposed to those who lived sedentary lifestyles (Rigby & Wright, 2020).

Brisk Walking

Loretta DiPietro, Professor of Exercise and Nutrition Sciences at George Washington University's Milken Institute School of Public Health, co-authored a small walking-gut study. Outcomes showed that walking for 15 minutes after food consumption reduced the blood glucose spikes of older adults with type 2 diabetes. Short after-dinner walks, according to the research team, help regulate blood sugar faster than mid-morning or late-afternoon walks. Since exercise may provoke peristalsis (food transit time via the GI tract), Sheri Colberg-Ochs, Professor Emerita of Exercise Science, Old Dominion University, confirmed that post-meal walks aid more effective blood sugar regulation than the pre-meal option (Heid, 2018).

A 2017 comparative review evaluated the impacts of brisk walking on middle-aged, overweight women with severe constipation. The participants formed two groups. While one group had 60 minutes of brisk walking three times each day, the second group didn't engage in any walking. The constipation symptoms of the brisk-walking group improved. Another study found that brisk walking could strengthen Bacteroides and other health-improving bacteria (Bumgardner, 2021). Other benefits of post-meal walking may include:

- **Decreases Gas and Bloating**: A 2020 review found that brisk walking, like other moderate daily workouts, helps improve bloating and gas symptoms in individuals with IBS (irritable bowel syndrome) by 50 percent. As we move, our digestive system is stimulated, aiding swift food passage (Palladino, 2021).
- **Supports Mental Health**: If you want to enhance your mental health, regular walking helps, because it decreases cortisol, adrenaline, and other stress hormones. When we walk, our body releases painkiller hormones like endorphins. Endorphins can improve mood, induce relaxation feelings, and reduce discomfort.
- **Boosts Sleep**: Regular exercise is an effective insomnia antidote. One study found that brisk walking aided sleep in older adults. A leisurely walk can also help induce deep sleep in individuals without insomnia.
- **Regulates Blood Pressure**: Brisk walking can improve heart health and prevent stroke, since it helps decrease LDL cholesterol and blood pressure. Individuals who undergo moderate-intensity workouts for 30 minutes five days a week may experience optimal heart health (Palladino, 2021).

Crunches

Since crunches prioritize the abdominal region, they help improve overall digestion. Crunches come in different varieties and creative exercise routines to prevent boredom. However, for optimal gut well-being, try reverse, vertical leg, or long arm crunches.

Crunches consolidate abdominal tissues and eliminate belly fat, a significant inflammation trigger. Curtailing inflammation helps improve gut health and activities and also prevents bloating, gas, and other digestive problems.

Whatever crunch type you choose, staying comfortable is important. Using your core to lift the upper body helps prevent the neck or head from injury. Keep your movements slow and controlled. Quick movement does not benefit the right stomach muscles.

Placing hands over the head during sit-ups or crunches may work for specific individuals, but if you haven't fully mastered this process, wrapping your hands over your head may weaken or hurt your neck.

Yoga

Some people love yoga because of asana, its physical practice, while others think yoga represents everything they hold dear in life. Regardless of your perspective on yoga, the truth is that exercise can improve gut health. If you want to keep fit, eliminate digestive issues, or maintain a healthy gut, practicing yoga can help, but always consult your medical practitioner if you have any doubts about such physical activity.

Yoga is an ancient practice with a wide range of physical and mental health benefits. It can help improve digestion, promote healthy gut bacteria, reduce inflammation, and even help with weight loss. Not only does yoga provide physical benefits such as increased flexibility, strength, and balance, but the calming effects of its breathing exercises can also soothe the mind and support mental well-being.

Studies have revealed that regular yoga practice can reduce symptoms related to digestive issues like irritable bowel syndrome (IBS) and acid reflux (Kavuri et al., 2015). This is believed to be due to improved muscular control from learning proper posture during poses, as well as improved stress management through meditation and relaxation techniques. Additionally, yoga's deep breathing technique helps stimulate the parasympathetic nervous system, which is responsible for slowing down digestion. It has also been suggested that certain poses in yoga may aid in releasing gas from constipation or bloating.

A promising study by the journal *Frontiers in Psychiatry* in 2018 has demonstrated that a combination of yoga and meditation can alleviate the symptoms of irritable bowel syndrome (IBS) and improve gut microbiota composition in women suffering from the disorder.

The study gives hope to people suffering from IBS, showcasing the positive effects of yoga and meditation practices on the disorder. In this study, women with IBS participated in a two-month program that entailed practicing yoga and meditation. The results showed significant improvements in the participants' gut microbiota composition and reduced symptoms of IBS.

By bringing attention and awareness to the importance of these practices in improving one's overall health and well-being, we could make great strides in reducing the prevalence of disorders such as IBS. Thus, this study provides further evidence that combining yoga and meditation with traditional medical treatments may be beneficial for those struggling with chronic health conditions like IBS.

Breathing is an important aspect of these moves and as a general rule, unless told otherwise, you should breathe through your nose. Sometimes it's okay to exhale through the mouth, though.

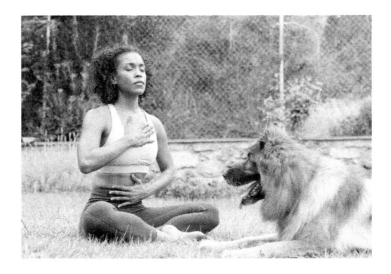

- **Pranayama (Breath Work)**

Pranayama aids digestion and also reduces anxiety. Depending on what makes you feel comfortable, you may do this yoga exercise on a chair or on the floor. Just follow these steps:

1. Sit up straight, shut your eyes, and position one hand on your stomach while the other rests on your heart.

2. Take a deep breath through your nose and exhale through the mouth. Repeat this three times. This is just to prepare you for the next stage.

3. Inhale through your nose until you feel your lungs are full, then hold your breath for 10 seconds and exhale through your mouth.

4. Repeat this six times.

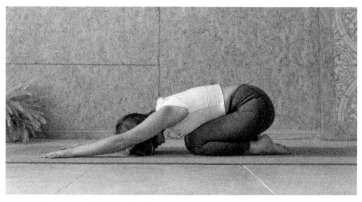

- **Balasana (Child's Pose)**

Balasana helps strengthen the digestive system. Make yourself comfortable by keeping your knees as tight or broad as you want. Positioning a blanket under your knees can prevent pain. If you have a yoga mat, better still. Follow these steps:

1. Start off from a kneeling position, sitting on your heels. With your hands on your knees, drop your shoulders and breathe in slowly through your nose. Without holding the breath, exhale slowly through your mouth.

2. Take another deep breath, then move your upper body forward until your chest touches your thighs and exhale.

3. Bring your arms forward, placing your hands, palms down, on the floor in front of you.

4. Lower your head and touch the floor with your forehead. If you can't get down this far don't worry, just get as low as you can.

5. Breathe in and out slowly, relaxing your body more with each breath until you feel totally at ease. Hold this pose for a minute or two.

6. Slowly return to the kneeling position by reversing the movement in step 3.

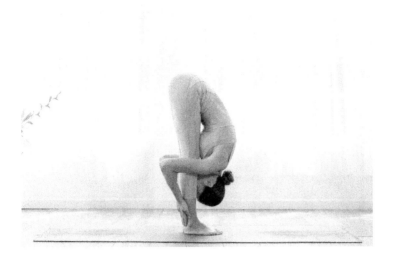

- **Uttanasana (Forward Fold)**

Uttanasana helps improve blood circulation and bolster the digestive organs as well as helps to relieve stress. It can be quite difficult for beginners, so you should adapt the exercise to suit your flexibility.

1. Stand upright with your feet close together, legs and back straight.
2. Take a deep breath and slowly exhale as you bend forward from the hips, not the waist.
3. The objective is to place your head on your knees, touching the floor with your hands, but if you find this impossible, you can modify your stance. Try placing a stool in front of you, reach forward, and grab the stool as low down as you are able, keeping your hips in line with your ankles.
4. Holding this stance, breathe in deeply through your nose and relax further into the pose as you exhale.
5. After about one minute, slowly return to a standing position.

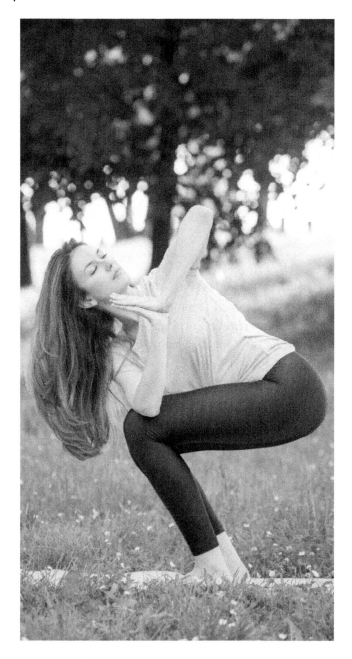

- Parivrtta Utkatasana (Twisting Chair)

Parivrtta Utkatasana can improve the body's mobility and act as a detoxifier. Feel free to take breaks, since this particular pose is a bit tough.

1. Stand up straight, toes together, heels slightly apart.
2. Bring your palms together against your chest, as though praying.
3. Bend your knees as though sitting on a chair and lean forward, turning your head to look over your left shoulder.
4. Twist to the right, moving your right elbow toward your left knee, and inhale through your nose. Exhale as you twist further, so your right elbow reaches the far side of your left knee.
5. Return to the upright position and repeat the process on the other side.

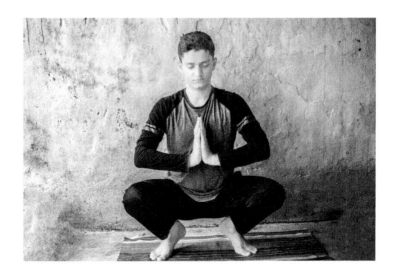

- **Malasana (Yogi Squat)**

Malasana strengthens your lower body, particularly your pelvic floor, and helps stimulate healthy digestion. This requires a lot of flexibility, so if you are limited in that respect, try sitting on a block or a low stool.

1. Squat on your heels with your bottom almost touching the floor.

2. Spread your hands, establish a prayer-like posture, and tug your elbows over your inner thighs.

3. Slowly inhale and exhale as you relax into the position, holding the pose for 10 breaths.

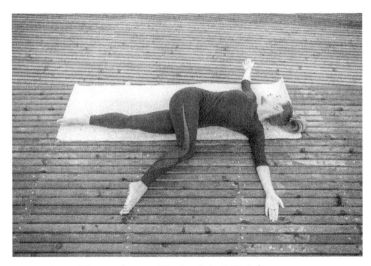

- **Supta Matsyendrasana (Supine Spinal Twist)**

Supta Matsyendrasana stimulates general body movement and acts as a detox. It is good for hydrating the spinal disks.

1. Lay on your back, pull your knees up to your chest and stretch out your left arm, palm upward.

2. Twist your body to the right side and bring your left leg over the right so it is almost touching the floor. Ensure that both shoulders stay firmly on the floor.

3. Turn your head and neck to the left, so you are looking towards your left hand.

4. Inhale deeply through your nose while relaxing your right knee, and exhale through your mouth. Do this five times.

5. Turn to the other side and repeat the activity.

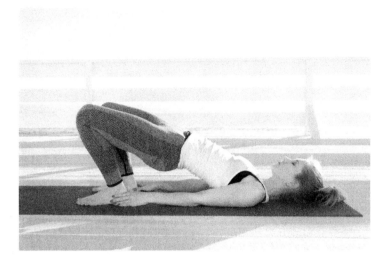

- **Setu Bandha Sarvangasana (Bridge Pose)**

Setu Bandha Sarvangasana can stimulate blood flow, which benefits the gut. It is best practiced on a yoga mat or a soft, non-slip floor covering.

1. Lay flat on the floor facing up, arms by your side, palms down.

2. Bend your knees and bring your feet towards your butt, so your fingertips are almost touching your heels.

3. Breathing in, lift your butt off the floor and thrust your pelvis upward. Hold this pose for a count of five.

4. Breath out as you lower your butt to the floor.

5. Repeat this for as long as you are able.

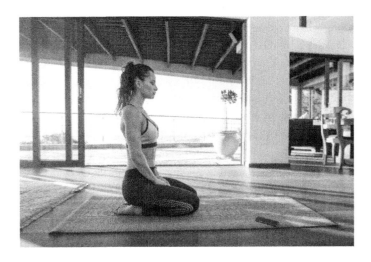

- Vajrasana (Thunderbolt Pose)

Vajrasana helps calm a person's mind, remedy digestive acidity and urinary problems, relieve knee discomfort, and bolster thigh muscles.

1. Start on all fours, knees and palms on the floor, feet pointing away from you.

2. Change to a sitting position, letting your butt rest on your heels.

3. Pull your ankles and knees together, edging your feet close to your legs.

4. Place your palms on your thighs or knees and move your pelvis gently a few times forward and backward.

5. Raise your chin, stretching your neck and lowering your shoulders. Breathe deeply in and out through the nose for one minute.

6. Return to the position in step one, then repeat as often as you feel comfortable.

Breathing Exercises

Everyone knows what it feels like to be stuck in traffic. Stressful circumstances often trigger fear, anger, and many other emotional responses. They can also cause stomach ache or increase your heartbeat. Stress hormones may trigger seizures or inhibit proper gut muscle functioning. Thankfully, breathing exercises can help us regulate our stress response.

Breathing activity can also improve digestion and help with GI tract troubles. Deep breathing aids relaxation, lowers heart rate, improves blood oxygenation, and stimulates concentration. Since deep breathing functions much like pleasant massaging activities, it can help calm bloating, constipation, abdominal discomfort, and other digestive issues. Breathing exercises for boosting gut health include:

- **Extended Exhale:** Inhale through your mouth and hold your breath for seven seconds before breathing out slowly via your nose five times. If following this routine looks difficult, try inhaling and exhaling two counts and four counts, respectively. Run the process for five or more minutes.
- **Zen Breath:** Inhale and exhale deeply via your nostrils, watching your belly expand and relax. Repeat the breathing exercise for 10 or 15 minutes.
- **Tension Release:** Lay on the floor, palm facing upward and arms extended at your side. Ease your breathing, relaxing your body from toe to head. If you feel discomfort, inhale and exhale deeply through your mouth.
- **Chakra Cleanse:** Sit up straight, legs crossed, maintaining an equal shoulder to hip ratio. Inhale deeply and exhale through your nose. This breathing activity helps ease tension, and may be repeated as often as needed.

Deep breathing, according to recent studies, can aid stress management, remedy or prevent chronic respiratory disorders, and boost digestion. Using deep breathing to soothe stress also improves gut health. Beth Chiodo, owner of Nutritional Living, said pre-meal deep breathing exercises can stimulate digestion, boost the vagus nerve, and regulate gastric acid secretion.

Both deep and slow breathing exercises can relax GI tract muscles, promote blood flow, and stimulate digestion, according to dietitian Mandy Enright (Manaker, 2021).

Case Study 4: Danny had been suffering from digestive issues for months. He was determined to find a solution and decided to incorporate yoga and walking into his daily routine. After 6 weeks, the results were remarkable.

His stomachaches had subsided and he felt less bloated after meals. His eating habits also changed, as he was more mindful of what he was putting into his body. Hunger pangs became less frequent and overall, Danny felt healthier. The physical benefits of the yoga and walking regimen were obvious, but it was the mental transformation that was even more profound. Danny began to feel calmer and more focused during his day-to-day activities, making it easier for him to stay motivated and on track with other goals he had set for himself.

The walks gave Danny an opportunity to clear his head while being out in nature at the same time. He took pleasure in breathing in the fresh air every morning before starting his day and found comfort in being able to connect with nature. The focused concentration he received from practicing yoga helped keep him centered through moments of stress and anxiety - allowing him to better manage emotions that could easily have overwhelmed him otherwise. By transforming both the physicality of his body as well as the mental well-being of his mind, Danny had made a complete 180 from where he'd started 6 weeks prior. He now had much more energy, and this carried over into all aspects of his life, making it easier for him to accomplish whatever task crossed his path!

7-day At-home Workout Plan to Boost Gut Health by Leaps and Bounds

Your gut keeps you healthy and comfortable. Presumably, you would do everything you could to strengthen and keep it fit, right? However, even if you eat a probiotic breakfast, drink kombucha for lunch, and avoid unhealthy food for dinner, you might skip a crucial part of the gut-health equation: exercise. But one recent study showed that individuals who did a 30-minute workout three times a day for six weeks saw an increase in their gut helpful microbes and had a significant reduction in risk for inflammatory diseases (WG, n.d.).

Committing to the proper exercise is crucial. While specific workouts promote a healthy gut or stimulate endorphin production, others hurt the microbiome. If you are pondering over what should be the proper gut activity, analyzing these expert tips can help:

- **Choose Low Impact (or Low Intensity) Exercises**: Integrating easy-on-the-body activities into one's workout schedule helps remedy GI troubles and improve gut health. High-intensity training can hurt your quads, hamstrings, and your gut. For example, Liz Barnet, a diet coach and authorized personal trainer, believes that high-intensity activity moves blood flow from the GI tract to the muscles, providing an athlete the energy to endure the exercise. So, as sweat runs over your face, your digestive system suffers, which may cause gut troubles (WG, n.d.). On the other hand, low-density workouts like brisk walking and yoga can boost direction and reduce transient stool time.

- **Do HIIT (High-intensity Interval Training) in Moderation Only**: High-intensity workouts do more than enhance mood or produce energy for the body. They can improve your gut health if you aren't suffering from any GI problems. Of course, box jumps and squats, like other high-intensity exercises, can provoke inflammation, so attempting excess HIIT can pose serious health challenges for those with gut permeability or other gut-related troubles.

- **Include Mindfulness in Your Exercise Routine**: Create a workout schedule that fits your condition. For example, you may follow a 2-day resistance activity with a 2-day yoga practice or a weekend-long hike. It all depends on what conforms to your plan. If you have an upcoming workout session, don't be anxious or dread it. Stress can aggravate GI issues.

Workbook Questions

Exercising your body is another strategy to improve your gut health and avoid digestive crises. Answering these questions will help you determine whether you fully understood the concepts discussed in this chapter.

- How does exercise enhance gut health?
- What workout options are safe for individuals who want to improve their gut health?
- What are the health benefits of post-meal brisk walking?
- How do breathing exercises benefit gut health?
- Why would one prefer low-impact workouts over high-intensity exercises when remedying gut-related health issues?

Exercise offers the gut many health benefits. It supports digestion, strengthens the beneficial gut microbes, and curbs many health complications. If you don't follow the proper workout, you will not realize the full extent of these health benefits. If you have any chronic conditions, seek medical advice before choosing a workout routine.

In the next chapter (and throughout Part Three) are delicious microbiome-friendly recipes that you can make at home.

PART III

MAINTAINING YOUR MICROBIOME HEALTH

9

BEST RECIPES FOR MICROBIOME HEALTH

Eating a balanced diet of vegetables and fruits helps strengthen microbiome health. These foods contain the essential fibers to increase and nourish good bacteria and improve gut health. For example, eating whole foods helps stimulate digestion. Emerging studies have linked healthy bacteria compositions to specific food classes and dietary structures. Diet is fast becoming a potent therapy for chronic conditions like IBS and ulcerative colitis. Read on to learn tasty and healthy recipes that could do wonders for your microbiome health and help you maintain an overall healthy gut.

Food Categories for Microbiome Health

Gut bacteria imbalance impacts several chronic health conditions to a greater degree than healthcare providers previously thought. For example, its diverse influence spectrum, according to recent studies, may include blood pressure, aging, anxiety, and depression. So, maintaining a healthy gut goes beyond improving your digestive health; it strengthens your mental and physical well-being.

Diet (apart from family genes, drug use, and environmental factors) plays a vital role in colon microbiota formation. For example, high-fiber diets can help broaden the beneficial microbes in the intestines. Microbiome enzymes facilitate dietary fiber absorption and fermentation to produce SCFA (short-chain fatty acids) for the human body system. These processes help reduce colon pH, the compound that determines the microbes that can survive in the stomach's acidic environment. Lower pH levels can prevent the growth of toxic bacteria (HSPH, n.d.).

Foods aiding increased SCFA levels include indigestible fibers, resistant starches, inulin, and pectins. These foods are called prebiotics because they are what helpful bacteria (probiotics) eat. Like many prebiotic supplements, seaweed, garlic, oats, Jerusalem artichokes, beans, bananas, onions, dandelion green, and asparagus are high-prebiotic food sources. The sudden introduction of prebiotic foods into one's diet may cause bloating or gas (especially in people with IBS and other gastrointestinal issues).

Laura Bolte, a researcher at UMCG (University Medical Center Groningen, Netherlands) led a team that analyzed the likely food classes and diets that primarily benefit gut health. The researchers categorized 160 dietary components under seven different food structures and examined their anti-inflammatory impacts on three primary participant cohorts – individuals with IBS (irritable bowel syndrome), ulcerative colitis, and Crohn's disease (Sandoiu, 2019).

Bolte said they examined the connection between dietary habits (or specific foods) and gut microbiota. The study aimed to demonstrate the effects of dietary patterns on the microbiome, because medical studies on this subject are scant. The participants filled out a Food Frequency Questionnaire and gave their stool samples to Bolte and her research team.

The team linked 61 different food items to 249 molecular pathways and 123 bacteria taxa. They also discovered 49 connection instances between food structures and microbial unions. For example, they found that enriching a diet with fruits, legumes, vegetables, nuts, red wine, low-fat fermented yogurt (or other dairy products), and lean meat could benefit the gut ecosystem.

The researchers maintained that plant-based diets could boost high SCFA production and strengthen the metabolism. Individuals with intestinal inflammatory conditions and ulcerative colitis usually have low SCFA levels. While plant proteins help stimulate amino acid and vitamin biosynthesis, excess consumption of refined sugars, red meat, and fast foods may provoke inflammation or reduce beneficial gut bacteria, explained the Bolte research team. Outcomes of this study showed that diet significantly treated gut-related health issues (Sandoiu, 2019).

Adopting the Microbiome Diet may help stimulate healthy weight loss and boost gut health. The eating plan emphasizes consuming particular foods and avoiding others. Raphael Kellman, a gut health specialist, developed the three-phase eating program below (Petre, 2019).

Phase One, which aims at replacing toxic bacteria in the gut with digestive enzymes and stomach acids, lasts for 21 days. Populating the stomach with probiotics and prebiotics and repairing impaired gut lining is the goal of this phase. This usually involves the Four R's strategy – remove, repair, replace, and reinoculate.

- **Remove**– Eliminate harmful substances, toxins, and foods that could accelerate gut imbalance or inflammation. Catalysts may include antibiotics, hormones, and pesticides.
- **Repair**– Consume more supplements and plant foods to improve microbiome health and heal the impaired gut.
- **Replace**– Eat spices, herbs, and supplements that improve gut bacteria and replace stomach acid with digestive enzymes.
- **Reinoculate**– Consume foods and supplements rich in prebiotics and probiotics to increase the healthy bacteria in the gut.

Avoid vegetables, dairy products, grains, starchy foods, and legumes. Other things to circumvent during this period are meat, fried and packaged foods, fish, fillers, artificial sweeteners, sugar, and fats. Eat organic and fermented foods like asparagus, leeks, garlic, kefir, sauerkraut, and kimchi. Recommended supplements include oregano oil, zinc, wormwood, vitamin D, and grapefruit seed extract (Petre, 2019).

Phase Two lasts for 28 days and aims to improve metabolism and strengthen the gut microbiome, making it more flexible in your diet. Keep the allowed foods in Phase One (but you may eat any prohibited foods three or four times per week). Your diet may include gluten-free grains, dairy products, vegetables, fruits, legumes, and free-range eggs.

Phase Three, the maintenance stage, does not have a time span (but you may skip it after achieving your diet objective). Your leaky gut will be completely healed, and you may eat 30 percent of the prohibited foods (except added sugar and processed foods).

11 Probiotic Meal Recipes

Gut health isn't just about healthy eating; it is about eating correct meals. Bacteria have a 1-to-1 ratio to human cells. In other words, we carry an equal number of bacteria as we do cells that make us human. Probiotics (the beneficial bacteria) improve mood, digestion, immune system, and skin health. Eating a probiotic-high diet is essential to gut (and overall) health. These recipes aren't just delicious; they contain tons of healthy bacteria.

1. Yogurt emanates from milk fermented by bifidobacteria, lactic acid bacteria, and other gut-friendly microorganisms. It helps strengthen bone health and regulate blood pressure. It also decreases antibiotic-induced diarrhea in children (and alleviates IBS symptoms in adults). Some yogurt products do not have live probiotics because they were processed, so be sure to request live or active cultures when ordering a yogurt product. Yogurt products labeled fat-free or low-fat may still contain high added sugar. Ensure you read the labels and avoid these, especially if they have artificial sweeteners.

2. Cinnamon Overnight Oats contain multiple live, active cultures and are super creamy. If you are looking for a fiber-rich, gut-friendly recipe for breakfast, you can't go wrong with cinnamon overnight oats. Spice up this delicacy with a bit of syrup, chia seeds, milk, and cinnamon, and enjoy! If you enjoy cooking and want to make this savory treat at home, assemble the following:

Ingredients

1 teaspoon of honey or maple syrup
1/3 cup oats
1/2 teaspoon of cinnamon
1/3 cup of Greek yogurt
1 teaspoon of chia seeds
1/3 cup of plant-based milk

Instructions

Combine the ingredients in a jar and refrigerate for 8 hours or overnight.

3. Kefir is a fermented milk beverage you can make using kefir grain and milk. Kefir grains contain lactic acid bacteria, and eating them helps strengthen bone health, alleviate digestive issues, and prevent infections. Kefir contains more yeast and beneficial bacteria than yogurt, and lactose-intolerant individuals have no problem consuming it.

4. Broccoli Cabbage Slaw tastes good and contains healthy, beneficial bacteria.

Want more fiber? Mix red cabbage with shredded carrots and broccoli before adding a lemony vinaigrette. Here are the ingredients you'll need to make your delicious broccoli cabbage slaw at home:

Ingredients

- 1/4 cup of olive oil
- 1 cup of mashed carrots
- 1/4 cup of dried cranberries
- 1 lemon zest
- 1/4 teaspoon of sea salt
- Black pepper to taste
- 3 tablespoons of lemon juice
- 2 cups of red cabbage – minced
- 1 tablespoon of maple syrup
- 1 tablespoon of apple cider vinegar

4 cups of broccoli – blanched or simmered

Instructions

Whisk maple syrup, lemon juice, salt, olive oil, and zest together to make the dressing, and set aside.

Mix cranberries, broccoli, cabbage, and carrots in a container.

Drizzle maple dressing on cranberry mixture and crumple to blend.

5. Sauerkraut, a lactic acid bacteria fermented shredded cabbage, has a sour, salty flavor, and it is pretty popular in Eastern Europe. Besides its fiber loads, sauerkraut contains high amounts of potassium, sodium, iron, and vitamins C and K. Its zeaxanthin and lutein antioxidants are good for eye health. Avoid pasteurized sauerkraut because it doesn't have active and live bacteria. Find the unpasteurized varieties.

6. Kimchi is a savory treat made from cabbage and other healthy ingredients like scallion, garlic, red chili flakes, and ginger. It contains a digestive system-improving Lactobacillus kimchi and other helpful bacteria. Vital nutrients one gets after consuming this goody include riboflavin, iron, and vitamin K.

7. Dark Chocolate-covered Blueberries is a gut-friendly, phytonutrient-rich snack you can make at home in five minutes! For this recipe, you'll need:

Ingredients

- 1 teaspoon of maple syrup
- 1 ounce of dark chocolate

Pink Himalayan salt

1 tablespoon of coconut oil

6 ounces of blueberries – fresh, washed and dried

Instructions

Melt maple syrup, dark chocolate, and coconut oil in a pan on low-flame heat. Remove pan from heat and toss in the blueberries.

Drizzle blueberry mixture on a sheet pan, sprinkle Himalayan salt, and refrigerate for 15 or 20 minutes.

8. Tempeh shares mushrooms' earthy or nutty flavor, although it is a soybean product. Soybeans have high phytic acid, the plant-based compound that impedes zinc and iron absorption. Since healthy bacteria ferment Tempeh, phytic acid is regulated to allow your body to absorb sufficient minerals.

9. Miso, a famous Japanese seasoning, is prepared with koji (a type of fungus) to ferment the salt-soybeans mixture. Other ingredients that can be combined with soybeans to make miso include rye, rice, or barley. Miso comes in different varieties – brown, white, red, and yellow. It contains many minerals, including copper, manganese, and vitamin K.

10. Pickles are tasty treats. Cucumbers are preserved in a water-and-salt solution to ferment, containing lactic acid bacteria and other gut-friendly microbes. Avoid vinegar pickles because they rarely have live or active probiotics.

11. Natto contains Bacillus subtilis, a beneficial bacteria strain that enhances microbiome health. You can serve this fermented soybean product with rice.

13 Prebiotic Drink Recipes

There are good microbes in our stomach that help to digest the food we eat and help absorb nutrients into our bodies. But there are harmful microbes as well. When the bad microbes take over, we experience bloating, headache, gas, constipation, diarrhea, and brain fog. So, keeping a healthy balance of the good microbes over the harmful microbes is very important.

How do you maintain good gut health? Probiotics contain strains of good bacteria and are often prescribed by doctors. Many prebiotic drinks are available on the market, but choosing the right ones can be confusing. Also, they are generally expensive. The good news is that flavorful prebiotic drinks can be made quickly at home using traditional recipes.

1. Beetroot Prebiotic Drink, a regular Indian beverage, tastes tangy but has several health benefits. To make this prebiotic drink recipe, you'll need:

Ingredients

3 or 4 beetroot – cut into strips
1 tablespoon of black mustard – crushed
1 tablespoon of salt

Instructions

1. Pour 1 liter of filtered water into a glass jar.
2. Stir in mustard.
3. Add the beetroot strips.
4. Close the lid with a cover or muslin cloth.
5. Keep the jar on the kitchen counter for five or six days. Open daily and release any gas formed.
6. Filter out the liquid. Store the prebiotic drink in a glass bottle in the fridge.
7. Save the beetroot to use as a pickle with your meal. You can drink one glass a day. If the taste is too strong for you, dilute it with water.

2. Really Green Smoothie is a creamy, heart-friendly kale and avocado mixture. It is loaded with essential nutrients, including omega-3 fatty acids and fiber. You can make this green smoothie at home using the following:

Ingredients

1 large, ripe banana

1 cup of ice cubes

1 cup of kale – coarsely diced

2 teaspoons of honey

1 cup of unsweetened almond milk

1 tablespoon of chia seeds

1/4 ripe avocado

Instructions

Blend the ingredients to make a creamy, smooth mixture.

3. Strawberry-Pineapple Smoothie is a nourishing and filling blend of pineapple, strawberry, and almond milk, and it takes just five minutes to make.

Ingredients

- 1 cup of frozen strawberries
- 1 tablespoon of almond butter
- 3/4 cup of almond milk – unsweetened, refrigerated
- 1 cup of fresh, minced pineapple

Instructions

Blend the ingredients in a blender to achieve a creamy, smooth puree, and serve.

4. Berry-Banana Cauliflower Smoothie is a thick, fruity, and healthy prebiotic drink, and making this nutrient-dense beverage takes a mere five minutes!

Ingredients

- 1 cup of cauliflower – chilled
- 2 teaspoons of maple syrup
- 1/2 cup of mixed berries – refrigerated
- 2 cup of plain, unsweetened almond milk
- 1 ripe banana – sliced and frozen

Instructions

Puree the ingredients in a blender for 3 minutes.

5. Strawberry-Banana-Mango Smoothie tastes great and contains gut-friendly fruits like banana, mango, and strawberries. Here's what you need to make it:

Ingredients

- 1 tablespoon of chia seeds – ground
- 1/2 cup of frozen strawberries
- 1/2 banana – ripe, frozen
- 1 tablespoon of cashew butter
- 1/2 a mango – ripe, sliced
- 1/2 cup of unsweetened, frozen coconut milk

Instructions

Blend the ingredients and enjoy.

6. Green Piña Colada Smoothie tastes delicious and is a blend of healthy fruits and vegetables. Here's what you'll need to make your super flavorful green piña colada smoothie:

Ingredients

- 1 cup of baby spinach
- 1/2 teaspoon of vanilla extract
- 1 cup of plain, nonfat Greek yogurt
- Coconut flakes – unsweetened
- 1 cup of frozen pineapple chunks
- 1/2 cup of coconut milk

Instructions

1. Blend the ingredients (excluding coconut flakes) in a blender to create a puree.
2. Coat with coconut flakes.

7. Spinach-Avocado Smoothie is a mixture of healthy prebiotic fruits like bananas, yogurt, and avocado. To maximize its nutrient blend, make your spinach-avocado smoothie and refrigerate it overnight. Here's what you'll need:

Ingredients

- 1 ripe banana – frozen
- 1 teaspoon of honey
- 1 cup of plain, nonfat yogurt
- 2 tablespoons of water
- 1 cup of fresh spinach
- 1/4 avocado

Instructions

Puree the ingredients in a blender.

8. Jelly & Peanut Butter Smoothie is loaded with lots of nutrients and antioxidants. Here's what you'll need to make this microbiome-enhancing recipe:

Ingredients

- 1 cup of baby spinach
- 1 tablespoon of natural peanut butter
- 1/2 cup of nonfat milk
- 1 teaspoon of honey
- 1/3 cup of Greek yogurt
- 1/2 cup of strawberries
- 1 medium banana – ripe, frozen

Instructions

Puree the ingredients and serve.

9. Creamy Strawberry Smoothie is a versatile, nutritious prebiotic. Its rich, creamy flavor comes from a blend of healthy ingredients like strawberries, yogurt, and honey.

Ingredients

> 1/2 teaspoon of vanilla extract
>
> 1 cup of frozen strawberries
>
> 2 teaspoons of honey
>
> 3/4 cup of milk – unsweetened, nondairy, and low-fat
>
> 1/4 cup of low-fat Greek yogurt

Instructions

Blend the ingredients for 3 minutes and serve.

10. Make-Ahead Smoothie can be a perfect breakfast treat for kids, and is a mixture of healthy, gut-friendly fruits. You'll need just three ingredients – blueberries, banana, and soy milk.

Ingredients

> 1 cup of unsweetened soy milk
>
> 1/2 cup of whole blueberries
>
> 1/2 banana – ripe, sliced and halved

Instructions

1. Combine the banana and blueberries in an air-tight plastic bag and refrigerate for 30 minutes.
2. Empty the contents into a blender, add the soy milk, and blend for 5 minutes.

11. Red Berry Smoothie is a healthy strawberry and raspberry mixture and a delicious breakfast or snack for strengthening gut health.

Ingredients

> 1 cup of nonfat milk
>
> 1 cup of chopped ice
>
> 6 ounces of nonfat strawberry yogurt
>
> 1/2 cup of fresh, red raspberries
>
> 1 cup of strawberries – fresh, shredded

Instructions

Blend strawberries, raspberries, milk, and yogurt for 3 minutes.

Add ice and blend for another 2 minutes.

1. **Green Smoothie**, a creamy drink with high omega-3 fatty acids, is suitable for microbiome health. You will need these to make your green smoothie:

Ingredients

1 tablespoon of ground flaxseed

2 medium ripe bananas

12 ice cubes

1/2 cup of cold orange juice

1 pear – mature, scraped, and diced

1/2 cup of cold water

2 cups of kale leaves – stem removed, rinsed, and shredded

Instructions

Blend the ingredients in a blender to make a creamy, smooth puree.

13. Whipped Frozen Pink Lemonade tastes tangy, but contains plenty of nutrients and antioxidants. You need these ingredients to make your nutritious lemonade drink:

For Syrup

1 lemon zest

1/2 cup of water

1/2 cup of granulated sugar

For Whipped Lemonade

1/3 cup of fresh lemon juice

1/2 cup of ice cubes

1 cup of unsweetened, nondairy milk

1 cup of frozen strawberries

For Garnish

Lemon slices

Instructions

(Make the syrup)

Steam sugar and water in a pan for 3 minutes to dissolve the sugar.

Add lemon zest, stir, and remove the pan from the heat.

Sift the syrup and refrigerate for 1 week.

(Make the whipped lemonade)

Blend the lemonade ingredients for 5 minutes to crush the ice and smooth the puree.

Combine syrup and whipped lemonade in a glass, and garnish with lemon slices, then serve.

All these prebiotic drinks help strengthen gut health.

8 Special Yogurt Recipes You Can Enjoy Anytime

Greek yogurt is trendy nowadays because of its abundant probiotics and proteins, but sticking to the age-old breakfast of granola and Greek yogurt can be irritating and exhausting. So, below are eight flavorful yogurt recipes you can enjoy anytime.

1. **Lassi**, a fermented yogurt drink recipe, is common in India. Lassi has different flavors (from spicy to sweet) and tons of nutrients and gut-friendly antioxidants. For example, Mango lassi, one of the better-known U.S. lassi mixtures, is a natural source of vitamin D. Dahlicious and Bio Green Dairy are companies that have other healthy lassi recipes you can find at local groceries and malls.

2. **Non-dairy Yogurt** is a nutrient-dense recipe anyone can enjoy. If the reason you aren't eating yogurt is that your gut doesn't tolerate dairy products, you won't have issues consuming this type of yogurt. Non-dairy yogurt is becoming very common, and you can use coconut, soy, or almond milk to prepare it. Prominent non-dairy yogurt varieties include Almond Dream, Silk, So Delicious, and Kite Hill.

3. **Tzatziki** is a nourishing yogurt-based sauce. It combines yogurt creaminess, garlic and fresh herb medicinal qualities, and lemon juice flavors. Whether you are buying already-made tzatziki or making the recipe at home, storing it in an air-tight bag ensures you have a healthy meal to last you a few days.

4. **Greek Yogurt Cheesecake** is an irresistible protein-rich recipe. Some people think cheese is used to make this creamy dessert, but that's not true. Greek yogurt cheesecake is a tofu and yogurt mix seasoned with vanilla extract, lemon juice, and maple syrup or honey.

5. **Frozen Yogurt** is available in many self-serve yogurt shops. Apart from its savory taste, frozen yogurt is filling and nutritious. There

are several mix-and-match toppings you can purchase to garnish it. Many food products contain frozen yogurt, as well, so check out the freezer section in your grocery store.

6. **Kefir,** a fermented yogurt drink like lassi, has a tangy taste. Although kefir has different mixtures, each variety has a unique flavor. Kefir became popular among Americans after studies showed it contains beneficial bacteria that could stimulate lactose digestion. Lifeway and Helios are common kefir brands sold in grocery stores.

7. **Peanut Butter Yogurt** is what you get when you mix peanut, yogurt, and almond butter. Peanut butter yogurt can be a perfect, gut-healthy breakfast when eaten with blueberries.

8. **Peach and Blueberries with Greek Yogurt Bowl** is a delicious treat packed with loads of nutrients. Eating this nourishes your body with plenty of vitamin C and gut-friendly antioxidants. The blueberries and peaches add extra spice to the yogurt. Want a chocolate flavor? Add cacao nibs.

5 Yummy Pickled Vegetables Recipes

If you are making vegetable pickles, cucumbers shouldn't be your primary ingredient. Whether it's celery or carrot, almost every veggie could create a juicy vinegar snack. Sitting your vegetables in saltwater overnight helps them ferment and load up tons of beneficial bacteria, the same process kimchi, kombucha, and other foods undergo before they're used as probiotics and to stimulate digestion.

Choose veggies, get enough apple cider vinegar, open your Mason jar, and store up your healthy homemade snack as we discuss the five pickled vegetable recipes you can make at home.

1. Quick Pickled Vegetables: If you crave a savory pickled veggie treat, make this. It is a healthy blend of gut-friendly edibles like garlic, veggies, and apple cider vinegar. Quick pickled vegetables may be eaten or served at a backyard barbecue.

Ingredients

2 garlic cloves
1 cup of water
2 teaspoon of kosher salt
2 cups of vegetables (radishes, green beans, cucumbers, carrots, or jalapeños)

3 teaspoons of granulated sugar

4 sprigs of dill

1 cup of apple cider vinegar

Instructions

1. Rinse and cut the veggies (or trim the edges of your green beans).

2. Simmer apple cider vinegar, sugar, water, and salt in a saucepan and pour the contents into your Mason jars.

3. Combine dill, veggies, garlic, and other ingredients in the jars.

4. Submerge the vegetables with a vinegar-water mixture and put the lids on the jars.

5. Refrigerate your quick pickled veggies. If you prefer them crunchy, eat your pickled veggies the following day. If you want softer pickles, refrigerate the treat for five or six days before consumption.

2. Pickled Red Onions: Red onions help transform a recipe's flavor, and they contain loads of nutrients. Since you need a small red onion to make this, using leftovers helps. Maybe you've made some pizzas, tacos, or sandwiches but are looking for the perfect topping; use this.

Ingredients

1 cup of white vinegar

1 1/2 cup of red onion – sliced

1/2 teaspoon of peppercorns

1 clove of garlic

Salt to taste

3 tablespoons of white sugar

Instructions

1. Scrape garlic and chop onion into small slices.

2. Combine garlic and the sliced onion in a ceramic bowl (or large glass container).

3. Blend peppercorns, sugar, vinegar, and salt in a saucepan, and stir to dissolve salt and sugar.

4. Cover the saucepan and simmer the mixture.

5. Pour the mixture into the ceramic bowl (or glass container), drenching the garlic and sliced onions.

6. Store the recipe in a non-reactive plastic, ceramic, or glass container. If you aren't using your pickled red onions immediately, you can keep

them in the fridge for three or four weeks.

3. Pickled Green Tomatoes: Lycopene, the substance that helps tomatoes retain their bright color, protects human skin against the sun's ultraviolet rays. Lycopene prevents cell damage. Tomatoes also contain vital gut-friendly nutrients like vitamins B and E. So, when you consume pickled green tomatoes, your body gets enough support to stay healthy.

Ingredients

30 ml of black pepper – cracked

2 ml of sliced green tomatoes

2 teaspoons of dried oregano

1/4 cup coarse salt

6 garlic cloves – whole or diced in slices

3 cups of white wine vinegar

2 cups of olive oil

250 ml of water

1 chopped carrot

2 peppers – yellow, green, or red

Instructions

1. Cut off tomato scars before slicing them into small pieces.
2. Lay sliced tomatoes in sheets and place them in a big glass or ceramic container. Drizzle salt in between the sheets. Wrap a kitchen towel over the container. Set aside the container for 24 hours.
3. Squeeze the tomatoes into a colander to drain the liquid.
4. Combine vinegar, yellow, green or red pepper, carrots, water, and the squeezed tomatoes in another bowl. Submerge the vegetables in the liquid. Cover the bowl with a dishcloth for about 12 hours.
5. Steep the vegetable mixture into a colander and cover it with a small plate (you may place a brick on the plate to add some weight). Leave the vegetable mixture for four hours.
6. Mix black pepper, garlic, olive oil, and oregano in another bowl and stir everything together.
7. Combine the vegetable and garlic mixture in preserving jars. Ensure that the oil mixture covers the veggies and seal the lid.
8. Refrigerate the jars or keep them in a cool, dark room. If you remove some veggies, ensure that oil covers the remaining vegetables.

4. Crisp Pickled Vegetables: This crispy, tangy veggie treat is delicious. If you want it spicy, marinate your veggies in a sugar, guajillo chiles, and vinegar mixture. Crisp pickled vegetables can be eaten as a stand-alone dish or combined with other meals.

Ingredients

3 cups of cauliflower florets

Boiling water

1/4 cup of snipped chives

1/2 pound of baby carrots – split lengthwise

1/4 cup of parsley – flat-leaf, chopped

1 fennel bulb – cored and diced into small matchsticks

Extra-virgin olive oil

1 bell pepper – red, chopped into small slivers

7 cloves of garlic – smashed

1 zucchini – sliced into small pieces

1 bay leaf

1/2 pound of green beans – slashed into chunks

1 tablespoon of fresh ginger

3 guajillo chiles – dried, seeded, and cut into slim strips

1 teaspoon of black peppercorns

3 cups of apple cider vinegar

1 teaspoon of coriander seeds

3/4 cup of sugar

1/2 cup of white wine vinegar

1 tablespoon of kosher salt

Instructions

1. Mix bell pepper, beans, carrots, cauliflower, zucchini, and fennel in a large heatproof, nonreactive bowl or glass jar.
2. Combine chiles and boiling water in a heatproof container for 10 minutes to soften the chiles.
3. Sift the chiles and pour them into a big saucepan. Add bay leaf, apple cider vinegar, ginger, coriander, 3 cups water, wine vinegar, sugar, peppercorns, and salt to taste. Stir boil to melt the sugar.
4. Pour hot chiles mixture into the bowl or glass jar, drenching the vegetables.

5. Cool your crisp pickled vegetables, cover the lid, and keep them in the fridge for three days.

6. Pour the vegetables into a big platter, and sprinkle olive oil on them. Coat your chives and parsley, and serve.

5. Vietnamese Quick Pickles: Many people love this snack because it contains nutrients and antioxidants. It is a kid's run-to-the-fridge delicacy, and some don't even wait until they're out of the jars before grabbing them.

Ingredients

I cucumber

Sesame seeds

1 cup of rice wine vinegar

I daikon – peeled

Salt to taste

1 tablespoon of sugar

1 carrot – scraped

1 cup of water

Instructions

1. Combine the vegetables in a large Mason jar.

2. Mix sugar, vinegar, salt, and water for five minutes (or until sugar and salt fully dissolve).

3. Sprinkle sugar mixture on the vegetables, drenching them.

4. Put the lid on the jar and refrigerate it for three or four days.

5. Sprinkle sesame seeds on the veggies and serve.

Case Study 5: *John had been living with the misery that was IBS for far too long before he made his way to my office. He was desperate for relief and as we discussed his diet and lifestyle, I could tell he was open to any advice I could give him.*

John had always been a bit of an experimentalist in terms of eating habits, but even this hadn't been enough to offer the relief from IBS that he was so anxious to find. We talked at length about the different types of fibers that are essential for gut health, and about how certain microbes can play an important role in gut health.

As I recommended changes that would incorporate these elements into his diet, John's eyes lit up with relief. Here was something tangible he could do to help himself – something within his control! While it can be difficult at first to find the right combination of fiber and microbes (microbiome) that works best for each individual, John put forth real effort. In time, he began to eat more fruits and vegetables rich in dietary fiber, such as artichokes, beans, sweet potatoes, apples and oranges, while also adding fermented foods like yogurt or kimchi into his daily diet.

John quickly found relief from some of his digestive discomfort and soon felt lighter, both physically and emotionally. With continued care for his gut health – including regular exercise – John has now regained a sense of normalcy he'd never thought possible before consulting with me. It's a reminder that sometimes the simplest solutions are often the most effective when it comes to taking charge of our health!

Workbook Questions

Eating the right food helps strengthen the microbiome. Avoid processed foods and drinks at the grocery store, since they contain excess added sugar and other ingredients that may undermine your health. Answering the following questions will show you fully understand the topics discussed in this chapter.

- What food categories improve microbiome health?
- How do prebiotic drinks strengthen gut well-being?
- Are there probiotic meals that enhance gut health?
- What yogurts can boost the microbiome?

If your job is very demanding, eating out often becomes inevitable, but you have the weekend to make healthy, gut-friendly meals and drinks. If something improves your health or makes you feel better, don't skip it!

FINAL WORDS

Caring for your gut health is akin to tending a flourishing garden. Just as a gardener carefully cultivates the soil, plants the seeds, and provides the right balance of water and sunlight, nurturing your gut requires a mindful approach to what you consume and how you manage stress. A well-tended garden blossoms with vibrant flowers and bountiful produce, while a neglected one wilts and struggles to thrive.

Similarly, when you nourish your gut with wholesome foods rich in fiber, probiotics, and essential nutrients, you lay the foundation for a healthy internal ecosystem that positively influences your overall well-being. By eliminating harmful toxins and mitigating stress through self-care practices like yoga and meditation, you create an environment where your gut can flourish, leading to improved digestion, increased energy, and enhanced mental clarity.

In essence, by tending to your gut's needs with the same care and attention as a devoted gardener, you pave the way for a life that blooms with vitality, harmony, and optimal wellness. With the help of this book, you can learn how to properly maintain your digestive system to stay healthy and prevent chronic illnesses from occurring.

Think of this book as your personal gardener for your gut – one that will provide all the information necessary so you understand what is going on inside, identify any potential issues, and know exactly when something needs fixing or replacing. Be proactive about taking control of your own internal environment by reading through these pages; with dedication and commitment towards improving gut health, you'll be able to start living a healthier life today!

To refresh your memory of the book and help you flip to the section you might need at any given time, here is a quick review:

As you probably noticed, this book includes three distinct sections. The initial section delved into the fundamentals of gut health, providing insights on how to assess the well-being of your own digestive system. In section two, I offered a comprehensive four-week plan, encompassing various activities and holistic techniques designed to enhance gut health. In the final section is an array of delectable, nutritious, and practical recipes to maintain a balanced gut microbiome.

Once you have grasped the key insights of this book, you will be able to:

- Understand the scientifically-backed perspective on the leaky gut hypothesis, its symptoms, validity, and underlying causes.
- Embrace a holistic approach to enhancing gut health, encompassing proper nutrition and adequate exercise.
- Follow a logical, easy-to-understand holistic nutrition plan that seamlessly integrates cleansing methods, healing and rejuvenation protocols, optimal eating habits, and exercise options to fortify gut health and overall well-being.
- Explore delectable food categories tailored for microbiome health, and indulge in gut-friendly recipes for probiotic and prebiotic meals and beverages that anyone can create at home.
- Devise and sustain your personalized gut health plan, and develop a deeper understanding of the ideal food categories for microbiome health and gut-friendly probiotics.

In this book, I have offered a comprehensive, scientifically-grounded exploration of gut health and how to overcome challenges in maintaining a balanced diet, as well as an array of delightful recipes for detoxification and sustaining a healthy gut. For those searching for information on digestive and gut disorders or innovative solutions to address gut issues without resorting to expensive miracle products, my hope is that this book caters to your needs.

You are now equipped with the knowledge required to maintain a healthy gut and lead a full life. With these powerful tools and insights at your disposal, you will triumph over leaky gut and other gut-related health concerns. My wish is that you will embrace these strategies for a healthier, more vibrant life!

Now, please find a carefully curated Gut Health Task Card below. This Gut Health Task Card offers numerous advantages by providing valuable guidance on optimizing your gut health through dietary adjustments and lifestyle transformations. By following the straightforward steps outlined on this card, you will be well on your way to enhancing your digestive system and elevating your overall physical and mental well-being.

If this book fulfilled your gut-related health aspirations, please leave me a positive review on Amazon!

A SHORT MESSAGE FROM THE AUTHOR

Hey, are you enjoying the book? I'd love to hear your thoughts!

Many readers do not know how hard reviews are to come by, and how much they help an author.

I would be incredibly grateful if you could take just 60 seconds to write a brief review on Amazon, even if it's just a few sentences!

Thank you for taking the time to share your thoughts!

Your review will genuinely make a difference for me and help gain exposure for my work.

Thank you,

Duncan

GUT HEALTH TASK CARD

(To access a free downloadable version of this task card, please click on the following link: https://drive.google.com/file/d/1ImcN9ibWIx-vzulEJuTEEfaYw09m-cHq/view?usp=sharing)

- Seventy percent of your body's serotonin and immune system reside in your stomach. One important reason to prioritize gut health is that almost all health problems emanate from stomach bacteria.
- A lack of fiber in one's diet is oftentimes the major driver for poor gut health. Poor gut health leads to inflammation, food sensitivities and other health issues. So please, incorporate high-fiber foods like seeds, vegetables, nuts, fruits, and oats into your diet.
- Check your gut health. If you experience lactose intolerance, food poisoning, inflammatory bowel disease, diarrhea, stomach upset, or other digestive issues, let a healthcare provider examine your gut.
- Choose organic foods over highly processed foods whenever possible.
- Take care to avoid sugary foods and artificial sweeteners.
- As a rule of thumb, it's best to avoid highly processed foods.
- Don't over-sanitize your environment. Contrary to popular belief, there is such a thing as being "too clean," in that your gut microbiome could be missing or severely lacking in the good gut bacteria that provide many health benefits.
- Studies suggest that gut microbiota deviations are one of the causes of intestinal permeability. Having a large number of diverse bacteria in our gut can help stop intestinal permeability (the breakdown in our gut lining) and thus stop leaky gut in its tracks.
- Detox regularly. Drink eight glasses of water daily. Drink herbal remedies like fennel, nettle, ginger and turmeric, dandelion, and lemon teas.
- Practice intermittent fasting and eat fermented foods like kimchi, kombucha, kefir, and sauerkraut—blend keto with your fasting.
- Improve your lifestyle. Manage stress. Quit or minimize smoking. Avoid leaky gut triggers like processed meats, gluten, artificial sweeteners, sugary beverages, and junk foods.
- Eat more probiotic and prebiotic-rich foods such as dandelion greens, Jerusalem artichokes, asparagus, garlic, apples, and bananas.
- Stay active—practice yoga, do crunches, go on a brisk walk, or engage in other low-impact exercise daily.

REFERENCES

Abdulla, H. M., Yu, S., Rattanakovit, K., Badger, C., & Rao, S. (2015). Small Intestinal Bacterial Overgrowth (SIBO) and Fungal Overgrowth (SIFO): A Frequent and Unrecognized Complication of Colectomy: ACG Category Award: Presidential Poster: 2396. Official Journal of the American College of Gastroenterology, 110, S995.

Ambarasu, R. (2020, June 5). *Types of GI Disorders*. Retrieved July 6, 2022, from https://www.starmedicalassociates.com/2020/06/05/types-of-gi-disorders/#:~:text=Structural%20GI%20disorders%20are%20caused,correctio n%20of%20the%20structural%20abnormality.

Ashraf, R., & Shah, N. P. (2014). Immune system stimulation by probiotic microorganisms. *Critical Reviews in Food Science and Nutrition, 54*(7), 938–956.

Axe, J. (2021, May 7). *Salt Water Flush Recipe*. Retrieved July 22, 2022, from https://draxe.com/beauty/salt-water-flush-recipe/

Baranda, A. (2018, December 21). *Legumes and Their Benefits*. Retrieved August 5, 2022, from https://www.foodunfolded.com/article/legumes-and-their-benefits

BBC Bitesize (n.d.). *What happens to food in your mouth?* Retrieved June 30, 2022, from https://www.bbc.co.uk/bitesize/topics/zv9qhyc/articles/z7w3gwx#:~:text=F ood%20enters%20the%20digestive%20system,soft%20and%20easier%20to%20 swallow.

Better Health (n.d.). *Digestive system explained*. Retrieved June 30, 2022, from https://www.betterhealth.vic.gov.au/health/conditionsandtreatments/digesti ve-system

Bumgardner, W. (2021, April 27). *How Brisk Walking Can Help With Constipation*. Retrieved August 14, 2022, from https://www.verywellfit.com/walking-for-your-colon-curing-constipation-3435138

Brennan, D. (2021, March 24). *What Foods Should You Avoid If You Have Leaky Gut Syndrome?* Retrieved August 1, 2022, from https://www.medicinenet.com/foods_to_avoid_if_you_have_leaky_gut_synd rome/article.htm

Burns, S. (2019, April 30). *Use Fasting to Reset the Digestive System.* Retrieved August 1, 2022, from https://wildfreeorganic.com/wellness/fasting-to-reset-digestive-system

Buschman, H. (2020, February 10). *Human Gut-in-a-Dish Model Helps Define 'Leaky Gut,' and Outline a Pathway to Treatment.* Retrieved July 20, 2022, from https://health.ucsd.edu/news/releases/Pages/2020-02-10-human-gut-in-a-dish-model-helps-define-leaky-gut-outline-treatment-pathway.aspx

Campos, M. (2021, November 16). *Leaky gut: What is it, and what does it mean for you?* Retrieved July 18, 2022, from https://www.health.harvard.edu/blog/leaky-gut-what-is-it-and-what-does-it-mean-for-you-2017092212451

Cani, P. D., Amar, J., Iglesias, M. A., Poggi, M., Knauf, C., Bastelica, D., ... & Waget, A. (2008). Metabolic endotoxemia initiates obesity and insulin resistance. Diabetes, 57(7), 1470-1481. doi:10 1038Carver-Carter, R. (n.d.). *Common Gut Health Myths Debunked.* Retrieved July 1, 2022, from https://atlasbiomed.com/blog/common-gut-health-myths-debunked/amp/

Chai, C. (2022, June 2). *Can Exercise Boost My Gut Health?* Retrieved August 14, 2022, from https://www.everydayhealth.com/fitness/can-exercise-boost-my-gut-health/

CHF (n.d.). *Top 10 Reasons Why You Need To Eat Fruit.* Retrieved August 7, 2022, from https://www.creativehealthyfamily.com/top-10-reasons-why-you-need-to-eat-fruit/

Ciccolini, K. (2018, September 17). *If Your Gut Could Talk: 10 Things You Should Know.* Retrieved June 26, 2022, from https://www.healthline.com/health/digestive-health/things-your-gut-wants-you-to-know

Clark, W. (n.d.). *The Differences Between Functional and Structural Gastrointestinal Disorders.* Retrieved July 6, 2022, from https://whalenclark.com/the-differences-between-functional-and-structural-gastrointestinal-disorders/

Cleveland Clinic (2019, December 1). *Lactose intolerance*. Retrieved July 6, 2022, from https://my.clevelandclinic.org/health/diseases/7317-lactose-intolerance

Cleveland Clinic (2020, February 4). *Colon Polyps*. Retrieved July 13, 2022, from https://my.clevelandclinic.org/health/diseases/15370-colon-polyps

Cleveland Clinic (2020, March 9). *Probiotics*. Retrieved August 4, 2022, from https://my.clevelandclinic.org/health/articles/14598-probiotics

Cleveland Clinic (2020, April 22). *Colorectal (Colon) Cancer*. Retrieved July 7, 2022, from https://my.clevelandclinic.org/health/diseases/14501-colorectal-colon-cancer

Cleveland Clinic (2021, May 3). *Inflammatory Bowel Disease (Overview)*. Retrieved July 14, 2022, from https://my.clevelandclinic.org/health/diseases/15587-inflammatory-bowel-disease-overview

Cleveland Clinic (2021, October 13). *Pharynx (Throat)*. Retrieved June 30, 2022, from https://my.clevelandclinic.org/health/body/21869-pharynx#:~:text=Pharynx%20(Throat),including%20sore%20throat%20and%20tonsillitis.

Cleveland Clinic (2022, April 6). *Leaky Gut Syndrome*. Retrieved July 18, 2022, from https://my.clevelandclinic.org/health/diseases/22724-leaky-gut-syndrome#:~:text=Leaky%20gut%20syndrome%20is%20a%20theory%20that%20intestinal%20permeability%20is,letting%20toxins%20into%20your%20bloodstream.

DerSarkissian, C. (2022, February 20). *Leaky Gut Syndrome: What Is It?* Retrieved July 19, 2022, from https://www.webmd.com/digestive-disorders/features/leaky-gut-syndrome

Dix, M. & Klein, E. (2022, June 1). *Understanding Gut Health: Signs of an Unhealthy Gut and What to Do About It*. Retrieved June 26, 2022, from https://www.healthline.com/health/gut-health#improving-gut-health

Erdman, S. E. (2021). Oxytocin and the microbiome. *Current Opinion in Endocrine and Metabolic Research, 19,* 8–14.

Eske, J. (2019, August 20). *What is the best diet for leaky gut syndrome?* Retrieved August 1, 2022, from https://www.medicalnewstoday.com/articles/326102

Eske, J. (2019, August 21). *What to know about leaky gut syndrome.*

Retrieved July 19, 2022, from
https://www.medicalnewstoday.com/articles/326117

Foster, J. A., Rinaman, L., & Cryan, J. F. (2017). Stress & the gut-brain axis:
Regulation by the microbiome. *Neurobiology of Stress, 7,* 124–136.

Foster, K. (2020, January 6). *8 Filling Breakfasts That Are Also Good for
Your Gut.* Retrieved August 1, 2022 from https://www.thekitchn.com/8-
gut-friendly-breakfasts-22982178

Galloway, J. (n.d.). *3 Under-the-Radar Signs You Actually Have Great Gut
Health.* Retrieved July 8, 2022, from https://www.wellandgood.com/signs-
healthy-gut/amp/

Gunnars, K. (2020, December 9). *Probiotics 101: A Simple Beginner's Guide.*
Retrieved August 4, 2022, from
https://www.healthline.com/nutrition/probiotics-101

Health & Wellness (2018, June 18). *The 8 Most Common Myths About Gut
Health.* Retrieved July 1, 2022, from https://sheerluxe.com/life/health-
wellness/8-most-common-myths-about-gut-health

Heather (2015, November 22). *What's the difference between the terms: gut,
bowel, and intestine? Are they different?* Retrieved July 1, 2022, from
https://www.italki.com/post/question-
333275?internal_campaign=community_register_copies&internal_content=la
nguage_partners&internal_medium=pop_up&internal_source=internal

Heid, M. (2018, September 26). *The Case For Taking a Walk After You Eat.*
Retrieved August 14, 2022, from https://time.com/5405778/walking-after-
eating-good-for-you/?amp=true

Henderson, R. (n.d.). *The digestive system.* Retrieved June 25, 2022, from
https://patient.info/news-and-features/the-digestive-
system#:~:text=The%20gut%20(gastrointestinal%20tract)%20is,the%20back%
20passage%20(anus).

Hollander, D. & Kaunitz, J. (2019, August 30). The Leaky Gut: Tight
Junctions but Loose Associations? *Digestive Diseases and Sciences.* Volume
65, pp. 1277 -1287. Retrieved July 18, 2022, from
https://link.springer.com/article/10.1007/s10620-019-05777-2

HSPH (n.d.). *The Microbiome.* Retrieved August 18, 20222, from
https://www.hsph.harvard.edu/nutritionsource/microbiome/#diet-

microbiota

Jennings, K. (2019, April 26). *9 Health Benefits of Eating Whole Grains.* Retrieved August 12, 2022, from https://www.healthline.com/nutrition/9-benefits-of-whole-grains

Johns Hopkins (n.d.). *Lactose intolerance.* Retrieved July 6, 2022, from https://www.hopkinsmedicine.org/health/conditions-and-diseases/lactose-intolerance?amp=true

Johns Hopkins (n.d.). *Lumbar Spinal Stenosis.* Retrieved July 13, 2022, from https://www.google.com/amp/s/www.hopkinsmedicine.org/health/conditions-and-diseases/lumbar-spinal-stenosis%3famp=true

Kahn, A. & Jewell, T. (2021, November 8). *Causes of Hemorrhoids and Tips for Prevention.* Retrieved July 13, 2022, from https://www.healthline.com/health/hemorrhoids

Kavuri, V., Raghuram, N., Malamud, A., & Selvan, S. R. (2015). Irritable Bowel Syndrome: Yoga as Remedial Therapy. *Evidence-Based Complementary and Alternative Medicine: eCAM, 2015,* 398156.

Kleinfeld, H. (n.d.). *Can You Take Prebiotics and Probiotics Together?* Retrieved August 5, 2022, from https://www.omnibioticlife.com/can-you-take-prebiotics-and-probiotics-together/

Knight, R., & Beiko, R. (2010). Know thyself (through microbiome studies). Genome Biology, 11(10), 224.Kresser, C. (2020, June 25). *The 13 Benefits of Fermented Foods and How They Improve Your Health.* Retrieved August 12, 2022, from https://chriskresser.com/the-13-benefits-of-fermented-foods-and-how-they-improve-your-health/

Kubala, J. (2022, February 17). *You've Heard of Probiotics — But What Are Prebiotics? All You Need to Know.* Retrieved August 4, 2022, from https://www.healthline.com/nutrition/prebiotics-benefits

Lawson, F. (2018, November 29). *What Are The Best Foods For Leaky Gut?* Retrieved July 21, 2022, from https://healthpath.com/leaky-gut/what-are-the-best-foods-for-leaky-gut/#:~:text=These%20contain%20quercetin%2C%20a%20phytonutrient,essential%20for%20a%20healthy%20gut.

Lephart, E. D., & Naftolin, F. (2022). Estrogen Action and Gut Microbiome Metabolism in Dermal Health. *Dermatology and Therapy, 12*(7), 1535–1550.

Levy, J. (2018, January 26). *Is Coconut Water Good for You?* Retrieved July

21, 2022, from https://draxe.com/nutrition/is-coconut-water-good-for-you/

Lewin, J. (2021, July 29). *Top 5 health benefits of bananas.* Retrieved July 20, 2022, from https://www.bbcgoodfood.com/howto/guide/health-benefits-bananas

MacGill, M. (2020, June 4). *What you should know about diarrhea.* Retrieved July 7, 2022, from https://www.medicalnewstoday.com/articles/158634

MacGill, M. (2022, January 11). *GERD (persistent acid reflux): Symptoms, treatments, and causes.* Retrieved July 6, 2022, from https://www.medicalnewstoday.com/articles/14085

Manaker, L. (2021, November 19). *How Does Deep Breathing Improve Your Digestion?* Retrieved August 15, 2022, from https://www.verywellhealth.com/diaphragmatic-breathing-stress-digestion-5209648

Maphosa, Y. & Jideani, V. (2017, April 11). *The Role of Legumes in Human Nutrition.* Retrieved August 5, 2022, from https://www.intechopen.com/chapters/55808

Mayo Clinic (2020, May 22). *Gastroesophageal reflux disease (GERD).* Retrieved July 6, 2022, from https://www.mayoclinic.org/diseases-conditions/gerd/symptoms-causes/syc-20361940

Mayo Clinic (2022, March 5). *Lactose intolerance.* Retrieved July 6, 2022, from https://www.mayoclinic.org/diseases-conditions/lactose-intolerance/symptoms-causes/syc-20374232

Mayo Clinic (2022, May 10). *Colon Cancer.* Retrieved July 14, 2022, from https://www.mayoclinic.org/diseases-conditions/colon-cancer/symptoms-causes/syc-20353669

McAuliffe, L. (2021, December 31). *Leaky Gut Diet: How to Eat to Heal Your Gut.* Retrieved August 1, 2022, from https://www.doctorkiltz.com/leaky-gut-diet/

McDermott, A. (2019, March 7). *Do Saltwater Flushes Work?* Retrieved July 22, 2022, from https://www.healthline.com/health/salt-water-flush

MiNDFOOD (2020, July 29). *What is better for your gut: apple cider vinegar or lemon water?* Retrieved July 21, 2022, from https://www.mindfood.com/article/what-is-better-for-your-gut-apple-cider-vinegar-or-lemon-water/#:~:text=Lemons%20are%20rich%20in%20vitamin,and%20boost%20the%20immune%20system.

Mindd Foundation (n.d.). *Understanding Leaky Gut Syndrome and How to Heal Your Gut Naturally*. Retrieved July 21, 2022, from https://mindd.org/understanding-leaky-gut-syndrome/#:~:text=Ginger%20has%20been%20used%20for,leaky-gut%20or%20gastrointestinal%20infection.

Mudge, L. (2022, March 29). *What is gut health and why is it important?* Retrieved July 1, 2022, from https://www.livescience.com/what-is-gut-health-and-why-is-it-important

National Cancer Institute (n.d.). *Gastrointestinal tract*. Retrieved June 30, 2022, from https://www.cancer.gov/publications/dictionaries/cancer-terms/def/gastrointestinal-tract

NDSU (n.d.). *All About Beans Nutrition, Health Benefits, Preparation and Use in Menus*. Retrieved August 5, 2022, from https://www.ndsu.edu/agriculture/extension/publications/all-about-beans-nutrition-health-benefits-preparation-and-use-menus

NIDDK (2017, December 1). *Your Digestive System & How it Works*. Retrieved June 25, 2022, from https://www.niddk.nih.gov/health-information/digestive-diseases/digestive-system-how-it-works#clinicaltrials

Palladino, A. (2021, June 17). *Is it beneficial to go for a walk after eating?* Retrieved August 14, 2022, from https://www.medicalnewstoday.com/articles/walking-after-eating

Parkview Health (2022, January 18). *The importance of gut health*. Retrieved July 1, 2022, from https://www.parkview.com/community/dashboard/the-importance-of-gut-health

Patino, E. (2020, June 10). *9 Signs of an Unhealthy Gut — and What You Can Do About It*. Retrieved July 5, 2022, from https://www.everydayhealth.com/digestive-health/signs-of-unhealthy-gut-and-how-to-fix-it/

Pedre, V. (2022, June 21). *Exactly How To Use Intermittent Fasting To Lose Weight & Heal Your Gut*. Retrieved August 1, 2022, from https://www.mindbodygreen.com/articles/how-to-heal-your-gut-with-intermittent-fasting/

Petre, A. (2019, January 22). *The Microbiome Diet: Can It Restore Your Gut Health?* Retrieved August 18, 2022, from https://www.healthline.com/nutrition/microbiome-diet#:~:text=The%20Microbiome%20Diet%20generally%20encourages,wild%2C%20low%2Dmercury%20fish.

Petre, A. (2019, July 8). *What Are Polyphenols? Types, Benefits, and Food Sources.* Retrieved August 8, 2022, from https://www.healthline.com/nutrition/polyphenols#:~:text=Polyphenols%20are%20beneficial%20compounds%20in,heart%20disease%2C%20and%20certain%20cancers.

PHWC (n.d.). *The Best Things for Your Gut Health.* Retrieved July 22, 2022, from https://www.phwcbermuda.com/best-gut-cleanse

Pifferi, F., Terrien, J., Marchal, J., Dal-Pan, A., Djelti, F., Hardy, I., Chahory, S., Cordonnier, N., Desquilbet, L., Hurion, M., Zahariev, A., Chery, I., Zizzari, P., Perret, M., Epelbaum, J., Blanc, S., Picq, J., Dhenain, M., & Aujard, F. (2018). Caloric restriction increases lifespan but affects brain integrity in grey mouse lemur primates. *Communications Biology, 1*(1). https://doi.org/10.1038/s42003-018-0024-8

Pingel, T. (2021, March 24). *The Top 7 Foods to Eat for Leaky Gut.* Retrieved July 20, 2022, from https://drpingel.com/foods-to-eat-for-leaky-gut/

Pisharody, U. (2015, March 9). *The "Leaky Gut" Hypothesis.* Retrieved July 18, 2022, from https://blog.swedish.org/swedish-blog/the-leaky-gut-hypothesis#:~:text=It%27s%20used%20to%20describe%20a,blood%20stream%20to%20trigger%20inflammation.

Porras, A. M., & Brito, I. L. (2019). The internationalization of human microbiome research. *Current Opinion in Microbiology, 50,* 50–55.

Pratt, E. (2018, September 24). *Research Says Exercise Also Improves Your Gut Bacteria.* Retrieved August 14, 2022, from https://www.healthline.com/health-news/exercise-improves-your-gut-bacteria

Putka, S. (2021, May 17). *How Fasting Changes Your Microbiome.* Retrieved July 30, 2022, from https://www.inverse.com/mind-body/fasting-gut-health-science/amp

Rigby, R. & Wright, K (2020, June 16). *Gut health: does exercise change your microbiome?* Retrieved August 14, 2022, from https://theconversation.com/gut-health-does-exercise-change-your-microbiome-140003

Rodder, S. (2021, February 12). *5 foods rich in heart-healthy polyphenols.* Retrieved August 9, 2022, from https://www.google.com/url?sa=t&source=web&rct=j&url=https://utswmed .org/medblog/polyphenols/&ved=2ahUKEwjw9OO9p6b4AhUF7xoKHaILD FoQFnoECDEQAQ&usg=AOvVaw01Hphvy892e8MvxTMuJmY7

Rossi, M. (n.d.). *Gut Health Myths Debunked.* Retrieved July 1, 2022, from https://hcp.yakult.co.uk/news/gut-health-myths-debunked

Sandoiu, A. (2019, October 21). *Which foods are beneficial for a healthy gut microbiome?* Retrieved August 18, 2022, from https://www.medicalnewstoday.com/articles/326744

Schaefer, A. (2018, June 14). *Colon Cleanse: What You Need to Know.* Retrieved July 22, 2022, from https://www.healthline.com/health/digestive-health/pros-cons-colon-cleanse

Schwartz, M. (2020, September24). *3 Benefits of Fasting for a Healthy Gut.* Retrieved July 30, 2022, from https://www.health.com/nutrition/how-to-fast-healthy-gut

Selner, M. (2021, December 8). *What You Need to Know About Food Poisoning, Its Causes, and Treatments.* Retrieved July 7, 2022, from https://www.healthline.com/health/food-poisoning

Semeco, A. (2021, May 11). *The 19 Best Prebiotic Foods You Should Eat.* Retrieved August 4, 2022, from https://www.healthline.com/nutrition/19-best-prebiotic-foods

Shi, Z. (2019). Gut Microbiota: An Important Link between Western Diet and Chronic Diseases. *Nutrients, 11*(10). https://doi.org/10.3390/nu11102287

Shoubridge, A. P., Choo, J. M., Martin, A. M., Keating, D. J., Wong, M.-L., Licinio, J., & Rogers, G. B. (2022). The gut microbiome and mental health: advances in research and emerging priorities. *Molecular Psychiatry, 27*(4), 1908–1919.

Shroff, A. (2021, September 23). *Diarrhea.* Retrieved July 7, 2022, from https://www.webmd.com/digestive-disorders/digestive-diseases-diarrhea

Silver, N. (2022, January 21). *A Guide to Functional Gastrointestinal Disorders.* Retrieved July 6, 2022, from https://www.healthline.com/health/digestive-health/functional-gastrointestinal-disorder

Sissons, B. (2019, February 13). *Top 12 healthful fruits.* Retrieved August 7, 2022, from https://www.medicalnewstoday.com/articles/324431#:~:text=Fruits%20are%20an%20excellent%20source,cancer%2C%20inflammation%2C%20and%20diabetes.

Smith, D. (2015, November 22). *What's the difference between the terms: gut, bowel, and intestine? Are they different?* Retrieved July 1, 2022, from https://www.italki.com/post/question-333275?internal_campaign=community_register_copies&internal_content=language_partners&internal_medium=pop_up&internal_source=internal

Sullivan, K. (2021, December 22). *U.S. death rate soared 17 percent in 2020, final CDC mortality report concludes.* Retrieved July 14, 2022, from https://www.google.com/amp/s/www.nbcnews.com/news/amp/rcna9527

Ülger, T; Songur, A; Çırak, O; & Çakıroğlu, F. (2018, February 5). *Role of Vegetables in Human Nutrition and Disease Prevention.* Retrieved August 5, 2022, from https://www.intechopen.com/chapters/61691

UMHS (n.d.). *Your digestive system.* Retrieved June 30, 2022, from https://www.uofmhealth.org/conditions-treatments/digestive-and-liver-health/your-digestive-system#:~:text=Digestion%20starts%20in%20the%20mouth,moves%20food%20into%20the%20stomach.

Unbound Wellness (2017, November 1). 4 Ways to Test Your Gut Health. Retrieved July 8, 2022, from https://unboundwellness.com/4-ways-test-gut-health/

Urology Care (n.d.). *Urethral Stricture Disease.* Retrieved July 13, 2022, from https://www.urologyhealth.org/urology-a-z/u/urethral-stricture-disease

Usuda, H., Okamoto, T., & Wada, K. (2021). Leaky Gut: Effect of Dietary Fiber and Fats on Microbiome and Intestinal Barrier. *International Journal of Molecular Sciences, 22*(14). https://doi.org/10.3390/ijms22147613

Vetter, C. (2022, March 9). *Can intermittent fasting improve your gut health?* Retrieved July 30, 2022, from https://joinzoe.com/learn/intermittent-fasting-gut-health.amp

Viome Blog (n.d.). *14 Surprising Things You Didn't Know About Your Gut*

Microbiome. Retrieved July 16, 2022, from https://www.viome.com/blog/14-surprising-things-you-didnt-know-about-your-gut-microbiome

Wahowiak, L. (2022, May 11). *A Complete Guide to Prebiotics and What They Do.* Retrieved August 4, 2022, from https://www.everydayhealth.com/diet-nutrition/a-complete-guide-to-prebiotics-and-what-they-do/

WebMD (2020, September 19). *Health Benefits of Vegetables.* Retrieved August 5, 2022, from https://www.webmd.com/diet/health-benefits-vegetables#:~:text=Vegetables%20are%20a%20good%20source,raise%20your%20daily%20energy%20levels.

WebMD (2020, December 17). How Your Gut Health Affects Your Whole Body. Retrieved June 27, 2022, from https://www.webmd.com/digestive-disorders/ss/slideshow-how-gut-health-affects-whole-body

Wedro, B. (2022, March 18). *Food Poisoning: Symptoms, Duration, Types, & Treatment.* Retrieved July 7, 2022, from https://www.medicinenet.com/food_poisoning/article.htm

Wentz, I. (2021, September 1). *6 Root Causes Behind Leaky Gut and Autoimmunity.* Retrieved July 19, 2022, from https://thyroidpharmacist.com/articles/root-causes-leaky-gut-and-autoimmunity/

WG (n.d.). *This Is What a Week of Workouts Should Look Like If You Want to Optimize Your Gut Health.* Retrieved August 15, 2022, from https://www.wellandgood.com/digestive-health-exercise-renew-life/amp/

White, A. (2022, May 16). *How to Do a Natural Colon Cleanse at Home.* Retrieved July 22, 2022, from https://www.healthline.com/health/natural-colon-cleanse

Zhang, Y., Lang, R., Guo, S., Luo, X., Li, H., Liu, C., Dong, W., Bao, C., & Yu, Y. (2022). Intestinal microbiota and melatonin in the treatment of secondary injury and complications after spinal cord injury. *Frontiers in Neuroscience, 16,* 981772.

Zoe (2021, May 20). *Gut health check: 5 signs of a healthy gut.* Retrieved July 8, 2022, from https://joinzoe.com/post/5-healthy-gut-signs

Printed in Great Britain
by Amazon

50674492R00091